THE
MAN'S HEALTH
SOURCEBOOK

THE
MAN'S HEALTH
SOURCEBOOK

Second Edition

Alfred M. Dashe, M.D., F.A.C.P.

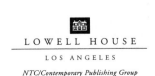

LOWELL HOUSE

LOS ANGELES

NTC/Contemporary Publishing Group

Library of Congress Cataloging-in-Publication Data

Dashe, Alfred M.
    The man's health sourcebook / Alfred M. Dashe. — 2nd ed.
        p.   cm.
    Includes bibliographical references and index.
    ISBN 0-7373-0109-0
    1. Men—Health and hygiene. 2. Men—Diseases. I. Title.
RA777.8.D375   1999
613'.04234—dc21   99-43149
                                                                CIP

Design by Mary Ballachino/Merrimac Design

Published by Lowell House
A division of NTC/Contemporary Publishing Group, Inc.
4255 West Touhy Avenue, Lincolnwood (Chicago), Illinois 60712 U.S.A.
Printed in the United States of America
International Standard Book Number: 0-7373-0109-0
99 00 01 02 03 04 DHD 18 17 16 15 14 13 12 11 10 9 8 7 6 5 4 3 2 1

This book is dedicated to my patients,
who taught me how to be a doctor.

Preface

In the several years between the two editions of this book, a few important discoveries have ensued. But for the most part, the usual pendulum swing between the discovering and debunking of purported miracle and calamity has been thrust upon us, as usual, by the media. Again, I urge my readership to take such information with, if not a grain of salt, at least a dose of calm.

Science does stride on, and some real discoveries, mostly in the "potentially useful" category, have been made. The Viagra® revolution springs to mind. A few other solid, therapeutic advances were made and most will be dealt with in this revised sourcebook. But for the most part, *plus ça change, plus c'est la même chose*—man's anatomy and physiology have not been altered.

A few good and bad news areas bear special note. First, the bad news: AIDS, which seemingly was beginning to show evidence of a cure, at least in some people, now seems to be returning in its full viciousness, even in some of the previously hoped "cured" individuals. Worldwide it seems to be the most threatening plague in current history, that is if biological warfare (or terrorism) is kept in check, heaven help us.

Also, we are beginning to see increasing antibiotic resistance of many disease germs, largely our own doing, because disease organisms have learned to cope with these human armamentaria.

On the good news side: we are getting better at prevention and treatment of cardiovascular disease and learning more and more about its causative factors.

Molecular therapeutics, or gene therapy, remains an exceedingly promising field at this point. We are beginning to learn how to insert helpful genes into deficient cells as well as perhaps how to turn off disease-causing ones. This, too, is for the future; not so far away, I think.

In my view, the most alarming changes that seem apparent are in the socioeconomic aspects of medical care in this country. More and more people are becoming uninsured and unable to pay for the care they need. Managed care, mostly profit-driven, is failing to provide an adequate medical system, resulting in angry patients and disgruntled physicians. A fundamental change in our health-care system is required—sooner rather than later, I hope. It's a view shared by liberal and conservative groups alike. We deserve better than we have, and we can get it, provided the leadership is there.

In any case, herbal magic is not the answer.

Contents

Introduction

Several years ago, while enjoying a brief working vacation as a cruise-ship doctor, I received a frantic 3:00 A.M. call. A husband and wife had brought with them a six-month-old baby. The baby was suddenly very sick with a high fever. This baby was, indeed, a very special one. She was conceived by in-vitro fertilization after many years of attempts by this now middle-aged couple. "What are *you* going to do about it?" they asked. I stifled my wonderment about what this family was doing on *my* ship on *my* shift. Instead, I attempted to reassure them with a recitation of my credentials as an experienced internist-endocrinologist and faculty member at a famous school of medicine. This seemed to rouse a response of incredulous fury. They asked, Why was I not a board-certified pediatrician, specializing in precious newborns? How dare I (with such meager qualifications) suggest treating this child? They assured me that the U.S. Maritime Service, the Navy, and the British Admiralty, among others, would hear about this.

It dawned upon me, almost as a revelation, how this dangerous conundrum could be resolved. I informed the folks, proudly and with sublime dignity, that I had raised four children of my own, all of whom were grown, functioning, healthy, and most of all, no longer living at home! They then accepted my services with nervous sighs of relief. I was permitted to see the baby. I treated her with some Tylenol drops which cured her and had her back playing shuffleboard in two days.

The point of this anecdote is this: I am not a (ahem) mere physician and professor. I am also a male human being, subject to all the pleasures and pains of this status. Also, I have managed to survive and function and I remain in reasonably good health, enjoying life. I feel perfectly justified in writing this book. It will serve, I trust, as a sourcebook of medical information about the adult male in health and disease. It is designed, as well, to be a guide through the confusing and perplexing world of modern medicine. Some advice, general and sensible, is given; of course, this is not meant to replace the irreplaceable—a competent personal physician.

When I accepted the challenge of writing this book, to be labeled *The Man's Health Sourcebook*, I was not sure what that meant. But I had occasion to mention the project to a number of friends—medical colleagues and nonprofessionals, male and female, youthful and not. The unvarying response amused and bemused me. To a person they told me that such a book about *sex* was sorely needed and I was sure to become a best-selling author. Not only this, but all, male and female, physician and laity, kindly and vociferously volunteered assistance. For example, "I can tell you about *sex* after seventy," (retired ophthalmologist); "I can certainly set you straight about male *sexual* hang-ups," (female psychologist); "I'll be the first to buy your book. I have a friend who has *this* problem," (barber); and so on and so forth. It occurred to me that perhaps men just might have concerns other than genito-urinary. Reproduction, after all, is the ultimate aim of sex, biologically speaking, but before reproduction must come production. The male genitalia (Kramer of *Seinfeld* calls them "my boys") require very complex anatomical and physiological support systems. So, although the "boys" will be dealt with at adoring length, it behooves me to discuss and describe the rest of the mechanism, in a systematic fashion. Please bear with me, or if you must, skip to the "good parts" and then go back.

The "health system" in this country is lauded, with some justification, as being the finest in the world. Certainly, medical technology has astounded us all, physician and layperson alike, with the fantastic advances of the past century in particular. These scientific giant steps have been logarithmic—faster and greater in shorter and shorter time. Contemplating this the mind reels. However, despite this we are, as a people, apparently frightened to death of living in what appears to be a terribly dangerous environment and time. We are whipped into frenzies of fear by media pronouncements of medical miracles followed in short order by medical calamities. We are frightened by our own bodies. For example, television often uses disease and disaster as a subject for entertainment. During the commercial breaks we are urged to use antacids, laxatives, deodorants, painkillers, antiseptics, and so on, lest we perish. This, despite the exhortations to indulge in the various possibly noxious beverages that are urged upon us to bring vigorous happiness and social acceptance on the beach. Even our food is touted as a healing medication. We are urged to eat right, diet, and exercise. We must eat popcorn for fiber, but *stop* eating popcorn because of the oil. We must take hormones this week for our bones, and stop hormones next week, lest they give us cancer. Honestly, what's a mother to do? What is the truth?

The truth is that miracle and calamity are both rare events. Most everything lies somewhere in between. There is a kernel of truth in most pronouncements. Personal health decisions therefore, if made wisely, will be made with cool objectivity and understanding of the facts, the theories, and the pros and cons.

In fact, we are an extremely rugged species and our bodies are tough enough to withstand many years of use and even abuse. We are living longer than ever (hence the worrying about the "graying of America"). If anything, overpopulation of the earth is probably the major problem of the future.

With a little bit of luck and some sensible measures of hygiene in our lives we, as average males, can look forward to seven or eight healthy decades. Even aging and dying can be healthy, as Dr. Lewis Thomas and others pointed out.

This, then, is what this book will deal with—information and practical discussion of the medical concerns of the adult male.

Doctor's Dilemma— Patients' Frustration: Why and How to Use This Book

Like it or not, the practice of medicine has changed drastically in the past decades. Medical technology and economics have been the reasons. Various diagnostic procedures, marvelous and unforeseen just a few years ago, have greatly changed the nature and cost of medical practice. Medical care, both therapeutic and preventative, has been deemed a universal right from pre-cradle to grave ("womb to tomb"). People are living longer and are creating an economic burden under which society is groaning. The cost of this is more than financial. Physicians have, unfortunately, been taught to use the laboratory to a far greater extent than previously. The time that used to be devoted to the face-to-face, doctor-patient relationship has shrunk to a fraction of what it was. The concept of "managed care" has descended upon us; that is, basically, an attempt to make the healing arts more businesslike and economical to society. The "doctor" has now become a "provider." A bedside manner becomes subservient to productivity. Health providers have been forced to compete economically as never before and fees now have been bartered down so as to make it necessary to increase the number of patients seen and to drastically reduce the time allotted to each patient. Patients are being forced by insurers and employers to utilize the most economical health plans, usually HMOs and PPOs and such, which simply cannot provide the personalized service of yesterday.

In one way, however, this may offer some advantage to the patient who is caught, as it were, by this system; health care has become incredibly subspecialized the past half century. Not only have the types and relative numbers of "specialists" increased, but even the specialties themselves have subspecialized into a maze of branches. The joke about the left-knee and right-knee orthopedist is no longer funny. An individual, unsophisticated in these matters, is truly helpless and in grave danger when lost in this labyrinth, with one specialist after another carving up the corpus. Under managed care systems, at least, the personal or primary care physician, usually an internist or family practitioner, becomes the "gatekeeper" and takes care of most problems, referring to specialists only when indicated. This gatekeeper, if well trained and motivated, will serve as the personal physician of yore. Having a personal physician with time and interest to give is still the most desirable type of medical care. Expensive care, but best.

In any case, it behooves the patient to become as knowledgeable as possible before seeing the doctor so that this precious time is better utilized. It is important to know what questions to ask (write them down before going to visit your doctor if you have to) and to have some ideas of the medical problems that one may face. The best relationship between physician and patient is one of partnership, in which questions are welcomed and answered freely.

This book is aimed to that end. The questions that have been asked of me in my years of practice will be acknowledged and answered in a systematic fashion. Often, the "answers" will be more of an explanation of the current state of knowledge of a subject rather than a rigid dictum. This, I believe, will be the most useful format for the reader. It will aid in helping both patient and doctor to get down to a more personal level in the shorter time that is provided for medical visits.

Incidentally, the book, I hope, will be read and enjoyed by women, too. It will be useful, I think, for those who wish to know a bit more about us, our concerns, our pains, and our little joys.

PART I

General Overview

Chapter 1

HOW TO LIVE

Luck and Risk

The greatest variable in a person's health is luck. There is little question but that one's genetic makeup is the principal determinant of one's future health. Of course, karma enters the equation as well. It is a good idea, for instance, to be born and raised in a solid family in a first-rate place. Unfortunately, little can be done to change one's luck, although the advances in human genetics and genetic engineering, scary and wonderful as they seem, presage the possibility that one's genetic makeup may be favorably altered. These are matters for the not-so-distant future, but already major social, philosophical, and practical questions arise.

In the meanwhile, since we cannot choose our parents, we can at least make use of the knowledge of our family health history, for ourselves and our children. For example, the presence of hereditary diabetes (Type 2) in our forebears, warrants nutritional and other hygienic measures which may forestall the "penetrance" of this trait. That is, we may have the gene but we do not manifest the disease, by avoidance of obesity and maintenance of an exercise program. We may avoid what appears to be a familial alcoholism trait by abstention. We cannot choose a place of birth for ourselves, but we may be able to choose, with luck, a safe place to live.

There is a long list of things to shun and it seems to be getting longer all the time. Certain items are noxious to begin with and are not debatable. Tobacco and illegal drug use, for instance, are generally accepted by all except the most cynical or naive as being suicidal habits. Less clear, however, are such items as the foods we eat, moderate alcohol intake, and so on.

Risk has always been a major concern of ours and more and more we face risky decisions. All of us make such assessments hundreds, if not thousands, of times daily. The contradictory bits of information that bombard us make the assessments more difficult, if not impossible. Fortunately, we have some help; seat belt laws, for instance. The myriad of regulations that exist in our daily lives, from traffic laws to the FDA, help decrease our risk burden, although sometimes they nettle and annoy us. Our perceptions of risk are colored and often overestimated by the dramatic and spectacular. The usual and far more common dangers get little attention because they are always with us. We in Southern California are terrified by the thought of earthquakes, but the mortality from these in the past twenty-five years is nothing compared to the deadly statistics of smoking and even unprotected sun exposure. In later sections, I shall try to point out some sensible and noncontroversial items of importance that will help define some of the common risks. In the meanwhile, stop worrying about meteor-earth collisions. For one thing, they are unlikely; for another, there's little you can do about them.

Of course, there are those who choose to participate in extreme activities—for example, skydiving, auto racing, rock climbing, and so on, which carry unavoidable elements of risk. These persons tend to be younger and braver than I. If asked my opinion of such activities, I will quote the statistics, see to it that participants are well informed, and wish them good luck.

Nutrition

Alarm, confusion, uncertainty, vague warnings, fears, and promises; all these are contained in the daily diet advisories thrust upon us by a merciless and mercenary media. Last night, for instance, the TV news anchorman breathlessly informed me that soybeans will prevent heart attack, cancer, and gout if only they don't cause goiter and kidney failure or acute heart failure from the salt in their sauce form. The bean is wholesome and nutritious but some strategy seems required to sell it. The only certainty in the matter seems to be that soybeans don't taste good to the American public! Just about every known foodstuff has received similar publicity. There is probably *some* truth to all these assertions; however, moderation is the key to nutrition.

There are a few facts that seem to have won consensus over the past fifty years:

1. Too much fat, particularly the (solid) saturated kind, is bad for humans. There is a direct correlation between saturated fats and elevated "bad" (LDL or low-density lipoproteins) cholesterol in the blood, arteriosclerosis, and cancer. The daily fat intake should probably not exceed 20 to 30 percent of the total calories eaten. Labels on foods can help in making this determination. Read the numbers and add them up.

2. We don't need as much protein as previously believed. Humans can get along with far less meat, milk products, and so on (which also tend to be high-fat carriers as well) than recommended previously by dietitians. Vegetable proteins, such as those in grains and beans, are safer, and the vegetables also contain fiber.

3. Carbohydrates, particularly the complex ones that are found in grains, vegetables, and fruits, should be the main source of calories. These foods also provide fiber, which is necessary for good bowel health.

4. Although certain foods have been touted as especially bad (for example, eggs) or good (for example, fish, especially for polyunsaturated fats), the evidence for these dicta is controversial. Better stick to moderation. Two eggs a week seems safe enough. If an egg, in all of its perfection, is bad, what on earth can be good?

5. "Natural" or "health" foods, generally, are usually of greatest value to their vendors. These soothing-sounding labels are no guarantee of safety. Remember, strychnine, arsenic, and cyanide are also natural

substances. The FDA has and will be further defining the use of the word "natural" on current and future food labels.

Salt and sugar are two very "natural" substances that have, in my view, gotten a bad rap. Sucrose, a simple table sugar, is simply a molecular combination of one fructose and one glucose molecule. It is almost immediately broken down by digestive enzymes and absorbed as simple, rapidly utilized carbohydrates—basic energy stuff. There is nothing unusually evil about sugar except that it provides "empty calories"; that is, no other nutrient value. Rapidly absorbed carbohydrates in *large* doses may be harmful to certain individuals (for example, diabetics, the obese, and hypoglycemics [those with low blood sugar]). Paradoxically, hypoglycemia may be aggravated because of the overstimulation of insulin production by glucose, which will subsequently lower the blood sugar. It is similar to feeding a bear; easy to start, hard to stop.

Salt (common table type, or sodium chloride) is the most plentiful substance dissolved in our blood and tissue fluid. It, therefore, is neither poisonous nor harmful when ingested in moderate amounts and is a necessary nutrient. The classic American diet contains an enormous surplus of salt over that which is required; about 10 to 20 grams as opposed to a 2-gram requirement for the average healthy adult. This is without considering the use of the salt shaker and especially salty foods such as pretzels, pickles, and the like. Some individuals with high salt intake may be subject to problems. People with cardiovascular and kidney disease may not be able to metabolize or excrete an excess of salt and may, therefore, experience salty fluid retention and circulatory overload (for example, congestive heart failure). Certain, but by no means all, people are sensitive to salt overdose and will respond with blood pressure rises (hypertension). This problem occurs with fewer than 20 percent of people, but one should have some idea of one's blood pressure. Excessive salt is best avoided.

6. Alcohol is bad in excess but probably good for adults, in moderation. Statistically, one to two drinks of wine, beer, or other liquor daily

seems to correlate with improved longevity and decreased arterio-sclerotic disease via unknown mechanisms (the "French Paradox"). This may be achieved by augmenting "good" (HDL or high-density lipoprotein) cholesterol levels in the blood. The "French Paradox" is the name given to the observation that French cuisine, laden as it is with delectable fats, especially the high-cholesterol type that is found in cream, meat, paté, and other rich, tasty, foods, has not killed fifty million Frenchmen by giving them heart attacks. Why? Could it be the wine, especially the red? A moderate amount of alcohol, particularly red wine, seems to elevate "good cholesterol" (HDL), which may have a protective effect. Indeed, the Framingham, Massachusetts, population study of habits and heart disease indicated that teetotaling may be as much a risk factor for heart disease as is smoking!

7. Starvation (generally fewer than 800 calories per day for an adult) for the sake of fashion or weight reduction is terrible for one's health. This self-imposed torture is relatively rare in males. Anorexia nervosa and bulimia are usually problems of young Caucasian women and are not seen in calorie-deprived countries.

8. Obesity is to be avoided—preferably by prevention (see next section).

Obesity

In China, the standard greeting is not "hello" but may be loosely translated as "Have you eaten your rice today?" Obesity is rare in China. Indeed, I was amazed to find, when making rounds in a Chinese university medical school hospital, an individual who had been hospitalized for two months, simply to evaluate his obesity. (His family was providing him with food, as is the custom in Chinese hospitals, but no one was monitoring the amount.) People in China and other areas where the population is hard working and calorie deprived do not suffer from the major nutritional disease of the Western world—overnutrition, or simple obesity. Arguments exist over the possible causes of obesity, but there is little doubt that the basic reason is too much food ingestion and too little energy expenditure. We, in the United States particularly, are blessed and cursed both with foods galore and energy-saving devices that have reduced our caloric requirements drastically. Some evidence exists for hereditary and other biochemical bases for obesity, but nonetheless obesity must always, in the last analysis, come down to eating more calories than one burns. This applies to all obese persons. Our medical-activist culture continues to promise easy ways to overcome this (for example, the recently ballyhooed mouse hormone, leptin), but all treatments that are successful must be so because either intake is decreased and/or calorie burning is increased. Perhaps, someday, a miracle medicine will be developed to accomplish weight loss without distress. In the meanwhile, we must work and suffer to succeed. This is no easy task with all the yummy food and drink thrust upon us ad infinitum.

Obesity clinics abound, many of them legitimate, some not. They must all depend upon the same principles of diet and exercise required to achieve the goal. The technique will vary, however. In the recent past, a popular method involved the use of prescription appetite-suppressing drugs, particularly the combination of phentermine and fenfluramine. Phentermine is related to stimulant drugs of previous years; dextroamphetamine and amphetamine, which are no longer approved for this use because of the addictive potential and serious side effects. Fenfluramine is mildly sedating and a less potent appetite suppressor. The combination seemed to help curb the appetite enough to permit some weight loss. However, these drugs had to be taken indefinitely. Since they were prescription medications, the patient had to be seen by a physician or in a clinic periodically, usually at considerable expense. If the medicine was stopped, the patient generally regained weight within a short period of time. Unfortunately, it was discovered after a year or so that some patients developed heart valve disease. This was serious enough to warrant the immediate prohibition of the combination. Some of the weight loss clinics have substituted another fenfluramine-like drug, Meridia®, which has been approved for use for only one year. Its effectiveness, too, has been questioned, as have other newer drugs, such as Xenical®, which block uptake of certain fats from food but which, unfortunately, may cause distressing side effects for relatively little long-term weight loss. Unbalanced diets fare similarly (for example, the Stillman diet, no-carbohydrate diets, protein-sparing diets). Such regimens are effective only because they are

---

Figure 1-1: IDEAL WEIGHT TABLE

MEN

HEIGHT FEET	INCHES	SMALL FRAME	MEDIUM FRAME	LARGE FRAME
5	2	128–134	131–141	138–150
5	3	130–136	133–143	140–153
5	4	132–138	135–145	142–156
5	5	134–140	137–148	144–160
5	6	136–142	139–151	146–164
5	7	138–145	142–154	149–168
5	8	140–148	145–157	152–172
5	9	142–151	148–160	155–176
5	10	144–154	151–163	158–180
5	11	146–157	154–166	161–184
6	0	149–160	157–170	164–188
6	1	152–164	160–174	168–192
6	2	155–168	164–178	172–197
6	3	158–172	167–182	176–202
6	4	162–176	171–187	181–207

Source: Metropolitan Life Insurance Company.

---

eventually intolerable enough so that total caloric intake is curtailed, frequently by nausea. Also, these diets cannot be followed indefinitely without serious nutritional hazard.

Why bother to avoid obesity? It has been determined, mainly via life insurance actuarial tables, that mild obesity (for example, up to 15 to 20 percent over "ideal" weight—Figure 1-1), may not be as deadly as once believed. Some authorities now prefer to use the BMI, or Body Mass Index, (Figure 1-2) rather than the old insurance company actuarial tables. This figure correlates better with actual body fat. Supposedly this figure, which is calculated based on height and weight, helps to determine whether you are at greater risk than "normal" because of excess fat. The calculation (use a calculator) is arrived at by multiplying

Figure 1-2: BODY MASS INDEX CHART

BMI Height (inches)	19	20	21	22	23	24	25	26	27	28	29	30	31	32	33	34	35
										Body Weight (pounds)							
58	91	96	100	105	110	115	119	124	129	134	138	143	148	153	158	162	167
59	94	99	104	109	114	119	124	128	133	138	143	148	153	158	163	168	173
60	97	102	107	112	118	123	128	133	138	143	148	153	158	163	168	174	179
61	100	106	111	116	122	127	132	137	143	148	153	158	164	169	174	180	185
62	104	109	115	120	126	131	136	142	147	153	158	164	169	175	180	186	191
63	107	113	118	124	130	135	141	146	152	158	163	169	175	180	186	191	197
64	110	116	122	128	134	140	145	151	157	163	169	174	180	186	192	197	204
65	114	120	126	132	138	144	150	156	162	168	174	180	186	192	198	204	210
66	118	124	130	136	142	148	155	161	167	173	179	186	192	198	204	210	216
67	121	127	134	140	146	153	159	166	172	178	185	191	198	204	211	217	223
68	125	131	138	144	151	158	164	171	177	184	190	197	203	210	216	223	230
69	128	135	142	149	155	162	169	176	182	189	196	203	209	216	223	230	236
70	132	139	146	153	160	167	174	181	188	195	202	209	216	222	229	236	243
71	136	143	150	157	165	172	179	186	193	200	208	215	222	229	236	243	250
72	140	147	154	162	169	177	184	191	199	206	213	221	228	235	242	250	258
73	144	151	159	166	174	182	189	197	204	212	219	227	235	242	250	257	265
74	148	155	163	171	179	186	194	202	210	218	225	233	241	249	256	264	272
75	152	160	168	176	184	192	200	208	216	224	232	240	248	256	264	272	279
76	156	164	172	180	189	197	205	213	221	230	238	246	254	263	271	279	287

Figure 1-2: BODY MASS INDEX CHART

BMI Height (inches)	36	37	38	39	40	41	42	43	44	45	46	47	48	49	50	51	52	53	54
										Body Weight (pounds)									
58	172	177	181	186	191	196	201	205	210	215	220	224	229	234	239	244	248	253	258
59	178	183	188	193	198	203	208	212	217	222	227	232	237	242	247	252	257	262	267
60	184	189	194	199	204	209	215	220	225	230	235	240	245	250	255	261	266	271	276
61	190	195	201	206	211	217	222	227	232	238	243	248	254	259	264	269	275	280	285
62	196	202	207	213	218	224	229	235	240	246	251	256	262	267	273	278	284	289	295
63	203	208	214	220	225	231	237	242	248	254	259	265	270	278	282	287	293	299	304
64	209	215	221	227	232	238	244	250	256	262	267	273	279	285	291	296	302	308	314
65	216	222	228	234	240	246	252	258	264	270	276	282	288	294	300	306	312	318	324
66	223	229	235	241	247	253	260	266	272	278	284	291	297	303	309	315	322	328	334
67	230	236	242	249	255	261	268	274	280	287	293	299	306	312	319	325	331	338	344
68	236	243	249	256	262	269	276	282	289	295	302	308	315	322	328	335	341	348	354
69	243	250	257	263	270	277	284	291	297	304	311	318	324	331	338	345	351	358	365
70	250	257	264	271	278	285	292	299	306	313	320	327	334	341	348	355	362	369	376
71	257	265	272	279	286	293	301	308	315	322	329	338	343	351	358	365	372	379	386
72	265	272	279	287	294	302	309	316	324	331	338	346	353	361	368	375	383	390	397
73	272	280	288	295	302	310	318	325	333	340	348	355	363	371	378	386	393	401	408
74	280	287	295	303	311	319	326	334	342	350	358	365	373	381	389	396	404	412	420
75	287	295	303	311	319	327	335	343	351	359	367	375	383	391	399	407	415	423	431
76	295	304	312	320	328	336	344	353	361	369	377	385	394	402	410	418	426	435	443

Source: U.S. National Institutes of Health, June 1998.

your weight in pounds by 705. Then divide this by your height in inches. Divide again by your height in inches. The result (typically in the 20s) is your BMI. The risks start climbing, statistically that is, when the BMI exceeds the number 27. BMIs over 25 deserve some action, if you wish to do something about your obesity. Incidentally, recent proclamations from the National Institutes of Health (NIH) state, rather too alarmingly I think, that the majority of Americans are officially obese. Longevity is probably not decreased much for most mildly overweight people. It is true, though, that those major killers of Western man, arteriosclerotic disease and diabetes, are directly related to increased body fat. The greatest burden, however, is social and emotional. Fat people suffer, especially the young of both sexes.

What can be done? Our aim should be prevention. Once obesity is established, it is terribly difficult to treat. Most victims find themselves yo-yo dieting, which results in major weight fluctuations throughout their lives. This is, it seems, probably worse for your health than staying mildly obese but stable. It is possible, and not unreasonable, with the aid of a physician and/or nutritionist, to maintain a targeted weight range as one matures. This may be accomplished, ideally, by avoiding excesses of high-caloric foods (especially fat and protein extravaganzas such as fast foods) and drink (especially alcoholic beverages). A regular practical program of increased activity is both extremely helpful and important. This does not have to be daily visits to the gym or aerobics. It may be simply something like walking to lunch or using the stairs, as long as it is habitual and pleasant, so that it will be continued.

In my judgment, the greatest hope for control of obesity, short of enforced famine, is keeping our children slim and trim with proper supervision of their diet and exercise. Once the age of eighteen is reached, a fit person may more easily remain so and may avoid the misery and unhealthfulness of obesity.

Vitamins and Food Supplements

My medical school alma mater, the University of California, San Francisco, has gained world renown for its contribution to the science of nutrition. Vitamin E was discovered there by Dr. Herbert Evans. Dr. Nina Simmons was instrumental in the discovery of vitamin D. The school was one of the few in the world that emphasized the importance of nutrition in the medical curriculum. Thus, it came rather as a shock and surprise to me as a young physician to find a lack of pellagra, scurvy, beriberi, and like diseases of vitamin deficiency in the general population. Only derelict alcoholics seemed to be at risk. As an Air Force doctor I was astounded to see in clinic healthy offspring of teenage mothers from benighted areas of the country. Some of these children were raised on fried potato sandwiches and Fritos given to them by their uneducated and poor parents. It seems that because of the nutritional discoveries in the early part of the twentieth century and subsequent federal laws regulating foods, vitamin deficiency in this country is a rarity. Our basic foodstuffs are "fortified" by government decree so that even marginal diets provide sufficient nutrients to prevent overt disease.

Indeed, if one eats anything close to a balanced diet, which includes grains, vegetables, fruits, and protein, malnutrition is almost impossible to come by. That is, unless one has a specific problem such as an inability to absorb certain nutrients from foods (malabsorption) or a special requirement (for example, pregnancy or diabetes). Overnutrition is by far the greatest public health threat. It is, therefore, unnecessary for the great majority of people to supplement their diet with extra vitamins, minerals, or high-protein "energizer" drinks. There is no scientific evidence for such a necessity. If this statement seems rash and bold in the face of all the health food and vitamin claims (and the billions of dollars spent on such) so be it! But, what if I am wrong and the vitamin promoters are right? What harm will it do to take these supplements? Most of the time, probably no great harm. If the money is spent needlessly, at least it is not going into weapons of war. Most (not all) vitamins and supplements are safely excreted by the healthy kidney and bowel.

There are some caveats, however. Some megavitamins are toxic in large doses, notably vitamins A and D and pyridoxine (vitamin B-6). Some amino acids (for example, l-tryptophan) have been shown to be toxic, and some herbal preparations are definitely dangerous.

Some vitamins and chemicals, commonly called "antioxidants" (vitamins C, E, and beta carotene), are currently under investigation to see if a purported anticancer effect may occur. So far, unhappily, the evidence is not forthcoming, but the studies continue. Prophylactic use of these substances has not proven to be harmful, so judicious use seems acceptable. Professor Victor Herbert of Mt.

Sinai School of Medicine in New York points out that these so-called antioxidants act as such only when taken in natural quantities that are found in food. He feels that the supplement pills are examples of "unbalanced biochemistry" and may, in such large quantities, be harmfully "pro-oxidant." Recently, the Physicians Health Study, which ended Part One in December 1995, concluded that after twelve years beta carotene provided no protection whatsoever against heart disease or cancer. Dr. Herbert feels that all supplements should properly be labeled: *Supplements can help some people, harm others, and have no effect on most.* I can't forget, however, that when I asked Dr. Evans in medical school (who died in his late eighties) whether vitamin E had anything to do with his vigorous and potent dotage, he winked wickedly at me and said, "Not on your life young man. I wouldn't touch that stuff!" The Physicians Health Study, which resumed in 1998, is investigating the long-term value of vitamin E and other supplements.

Exercise

We need to use our bodies vigorously to maintain optimum health; no question about it. We do not need to be athletes, professional or amateur. It seems to have been forgotten that Phidippedes, the original marathoner, dropped dead after his twenty-six-mile run just as he announced victory at Marathon. And he was a young, presumably healthy, Greek!

The problem for most of us is that we don't even walk, much less run! "Labor saving," a watchword for twentieth-century Western civilization, has taken its toll on our bodies and has engendered an overweight, unfit society. It is not likely that we will give up our cars or that the woodsman will drop his chain saw and take up his ax.

But, what does all this mean? What are the consequences of all this sloth and flab? We really don't know for sure, except that it is unsightly and somehow unseemly. It has not, apparently, diminished our statistical longevity, despite the exercise maven's dire warnings. Most health professionals will agree that a fit and trim individual will tend to handle disease better. Unfortunately, there is little direct proof that exercise, by itself, will ordinarily prolong life or prevent disease. If one is an obese diabetic, especially, regular and vigorous exercise may be very therapeutic.

How to Exercise

The term exercise means bodily exertion, which may be either recreational or work associated. Some lucky people have, by virtue of their occupations, regular built-in exercise and require no other measures. Two basic forms of such activity are:

1. Aerobic exercise—meaning basically, repetitive body motion such as walking, running, swimming, and bicycling, during which the energy expenditure and muscular utilization of caloric energy is just balanced by oxygen intake via the lungs. This type of exertion is thought to promote and maintain optimum cardiovascular (heart and circulation) tone and fitness as well as muscular tone.
2. Anaerobic, or intermittent or spasmodic exercise, such as weight lifting or most athletics (game sports) utilizes intermittent bursts of maximum energy and depends upon "energy" stores which do not immediately require oxygen for utilization. Anaerobic exercise is probably not as beneficial, although it may help to build certain muscle groups and may be more fun.

For practical purposes, it is important to remember a few points:

1. Exercise, to be of value, must be done regularly and habitually. The benefits are generally lost after two days of no exercise, and one's physiological benefits return to square one by the third day. Three or four evenly spaced days of exercise per week are necessary for maintenance.
2. Aerobic exercise may be mixed with the anaerobic type (via gym-type training) but either kind should be started gradually when initiated to avoid musculoskeletal or cardiovascular injury. Professional guidance may be advisable if one wishes to embark upon a vigorous program.

3. Vigorous athletics offer no known health benefits over the "low-impact" type. Walking five miles is just as beneficial and a lot safer than running or jogging five miles. Certain activities are particularly fraught with musculoskeletal hazard. Hence, the genesis of myriad orthopedic-sports clinics and hospitals.

4. Although various formulae for cardiovascular tone have been made available, such as increasing heart rate to a certain number or percentage over basal (a rule of thumb is: 220 minus your age = maximum heart rate; 60 to 80 percent of this maximum is safe), there is no strong evidence that this is important or advantageous over moderate, sensible exertion toward, but not exceeding, one's limits. Listen to the wisdom of your body!

5. Exercise programs and devices are notoriously relegated to closets and basements. The trouble seems to be a combination of laziness, distraction, and boredom. My experience tells me that a regular program may be achieved if the exercise is planned and pleasurable and boredom is reduced by measures such as sociability (for example, walking with a friend) or putting a TV or video in front of the ski machine or treadmill and watching *Good Morning, America* while "crossing the Alps."

6. There is good recent evidence that simply increasing one's usual physical activity on a regular basis, such as using stairs (whenever practical) rather than elevators, parking farther from one's destination to force a longer, vigorous walk, even fidgeting more when sitting, may have almost as much exercise value as the "official" stuff.

In summary then, healthy living habits combining moderation in food and drink, adequate exercise, and wisdom in risk assessment are, with luck, all that a person needs to stack the odds in favor of a vigorous and fit longevity. Sometimes, though, you need help from a professional. That's what doctors do.

DR. DASHE'S TIPS FOR HEALTH MAINTENANCE

1. The greatest variable in your health is luck, don't push it. Risk-taking behavior, such as substance abuse, is a common way to stack the deck against yourself.

2. Simple precautions, like wearing seat belts and helmets while in cars or on motorcycles and bicycles, will help put the odds in your favor.

3. Nutritional advice from the media should be taken with a grain of salt, and you should discuss any diet plan with your doctor before embarking on it.

4. Controversy rages on, but here are some good rules for eating sensibly:
   a) Fat should only be 20 to 30 percent or less of your caloric intake;
   b) You don't need as much protein as you might think, so you can cut back on meat and dairy products;
   c) Grains and vegetables (complex carbohydrates) and plenty of fiber will help keep you running smoothly.

5. If you eat a balanced diet as outlined above, you may be wasting your money with supplements of vitamins and minerals.

6. A small amount of alcohol, especially in the form of red wine on a daily basis, has been proven to help in the prevention of arteriosclerosis, but a large amount is bad.

7. Being obese is another way to stack the deck against you. It can lead to serious disease and premature death, usually due to arteriosclerosis, diabetes, and certain types of cancer. Weight loss through sensible eating and increased activity is the best way to lose weight, but consult your doctor about the right approach for you.

8. Antioxidants are still controversial in terms of disease prevention and longevity; fruits, vegetables, and grains are healthy sources of these.

9. A regular exercise program is apparently necessary for optimum health maintenance. Three times a week for twenty to forty minutes, whether it is walking, running, riding a bike, or taking an aerobics class, will help your overall health, if not your longevity.

10. Exercise is a great stress reducer, and stress has been a suspected culprit of many maladies. Find ways of relaxing and relieving stress that fit your schedule. Above all, just don't sit there. Do something!

Chapter 2

HOW TO CHOOSE A PHYSICIAN

According to *Men's Health* magazine, about one out of ten men have gone at least five years without seeing a doctor. Purported reasons include the costs in money and time and the belief that only the sick go to the doctor. Presumably these nine million American males are either busy or poor and/or well enough to meet these criteria, but at least some of them are making a big mistake, especially nowadays. Before the revolutionary Flexner Report on American medicine and medical schools in 1914, staying away from the doctor seemed the healthier thing to do. Survival rates for the undoctored were far superior than the "medicated" population. After 1914 things began to change. The break-even point probably was in the 1930s, with the discoveries of the sulfa drugs and antibiotics. Subsequent advances, particularly in early detection and preventive medicine, have made it clear that the physician has become an asset to one's health. The question then arises, what kind or type of physician?

Types of Medical Care

The choices are many and include traditional physicians as well as "alternative" medical practitioners. Alternative medicine is defined as techniques for treating or preventing disease that are regarded as unorthodox or unproven. This encompasses a wide range including naturopathy, chiropractic, homeopathy, herbal medicine, meditation, massage, and so on.

Allopathy

Conventional medicine, otherwise known as "allopathic medicine," has its roots in ancient Greek "physic" (or medical care) with Hippocrates, Galen, and others leading the way through the centuries—a most fascinating journey. Allopathic medicine is practiced by the conventional M.D. and D.O. (osteopath). Conventional medicine purports to be scientific medicine. It is based upon the rules and laws of scientific evidence as well as pragmatic (result-oriented) observation. The alternative methods of medicine are not as concerned with such rules, but are based upon results, often only of the anecdotal variety.

I am an allopathic physician and, therefore, my bias is obvious. However, allopathic physicians are pragmatic, too, and we have, over the centuries and now, subscribed to remedies that work even if we don't know how or why. Many standard medicines (for example, digitalis, ephedrine) are derived from folk remedies and were used for the result produced rather than the known mechanism of action. We must, therefore, accept the fact that some nonscientific healing methods are effective under certain circumstances and most of the time do no serious harm. If, however, a treatable disease goes undiagnosed and is inadequately handled by alternative practitioners, we, as scientific physicians, must protest and warn the public. Our physician-founder Hippocrates provided us with the first rule of medicine, *primum non nocere*—first do no harm, and we try. We must warn our patients and our public that the practitioner that attends them should be held to that same standard, at the least. (If not, they are merely shamans [medicine men] or quacks, as far as I'm concerned.)

How to Choose a Doctor

Assuming that an allopath (conventional M.D. or D.O.) is chosen as one's personal physician, the process of selection requires care. Much of the time these days the choice is dictated by one's medical insurance. Primary care doctors (or "gatekeepers") are usually assigned by the insurance company. For adult men, these will almost invariably be family practitioners or internists. If the former, the same docotor may attend your entire family. If it is possible, board certification in one of these specialties is desirable. Local medical associations may be available for advice, and local medical schools may be able to refer you to a list of voluntary faculty who are private practitioners. These doctors have usually been checked out as to their credentials and quality. I cannot recommend the use of magazine lists of "best" physicians which have been recently popularized. I have been amazed by some of the entries and I feel sure that some public relations personnel have been used to compile them. Advertising by physicians, once rare and considered unethical, is now commonplace and should be considered as reliable as most advertising. Sometimes, word of mouth from a trusted friend is the most reliable recommendation.

In olden days, before the Flexner Report, one could become a physician simply by apprenticing oneself to an established doctor. There were many diploma mills and unscrupulous doctors of dubious education who were only too willing to make someone a physician for a price. Standards and licensure were pretty much nonexistent. Since 1914, becoming an M.D. has been a time-consuming and difficult procedure requiring energy, aptitude, and strength (and financial support from some source). Licensure in the United States and most Westernized countries has strict requirements for education and postdoctoral training before an M.D. or D.O. shingle may hang outside the door. Usually, four years of premedical studies followed by four years of medical school, and between two and eight years of postdoctoral residency training is required. The residency length will vary depending upon the medical field chosen. Primary care doctors (usually family physicians or internists) need two to four years of training. Further subspecialty adds more years to the process. Medical schools are required to be inspected regularly and certified for accreditation by the various state licensure authorities. Foreign medical schools vary in quality but foreign medical graduates (FMGs as they are familiarly called) are required by most states to pass special examinations and take one to two more years of postgraduate training in an approved United States hospital before they are eligible for licensure. If it sounds laborious and tedious, that's because it is. One does not enter allopathy lightly these days, particularly since the economic situation has changed and immediate profound wealth cannot be expected by a young physician. That's good, too. We need physicians who are motivated by emotions other than greed.

A word about the initials that indicate professional status: M.D. = Doctor of Medicine; D.O. = Doctor of Osteopathy; D.C. = Doctor of Chiropractic; D.P.M. = Doctor of Podiatric Medicine (podiatrists); O.D. = Doctor of Optometry (non-M.D. eye doctor who is unable to prescribe medicines or do surgery). The following letters also may follow a doctor's name:

FACP = Fellow of the American College of Physicians
FACS = Fellow of the American College of Surgeons
FACOG = Fellow of the American College of Ob-Gyn

These fellowships are granted only to board-certified specialists in their fields who also have shown appropriate skill and knowledge for this recognition. Board certification means that specialty status has been achieved by the doctor by passage of certain examinations. Such a certification may be denoted by the title "Diplomate of the American Board of Internal Medicine" or "Family Practice", and so on. Do not hesitate to ask your doctor about his or her training or certification. If there is a question about qualification, the library has reference books listing physicians by name and specialty. I do not mean to imply, nor should you infer, that a recognized United States medical school and legitimate diplomas necessarily add up to a fine physician for your purposes. Quality and compatibility are determined by many criteria, but it is helpful nontheless to know your doctor's background.

The matter of the sex of your personal physician needs some mention. Women physicians now constitute about 40 percent of medical graduates in the United States. There is a tendency for women physicians to gravitate to fields that will permit them to have adequate time for family and child-rearing, so the number of female primary care physicians is relatively small compared to male. I believe that the choice of male versus female for one's personal doctor should be strictly based upon one's preferences and inhibitions. There is no inherent advantage or disadvantage in the choice.

Once a physician is chosen, a meeting is necessary to determine compatibility. This may be done as a brief visit during which questions and answers may be traded and patient and doctor may size each other up. Ideally, the initial meeting should be followed by a more or less complete history and physical examination, which is very valuable for the future medical relationship. The doctor will have some knowledge of the patient's basal status and present and potential medical problems. If none are present, fine. General notions of hygiene may be discussed and plans and recommendations for future evaluations outlined. The patient benefits greatly by this knowledge of current health and future potential problems. He will learn how much and how often medical care is warranted in his case and, most importantly, he will have at hand an obligated physician in case of emergency. It is difficult to find a new personal doctor in the middle of the night or on the weekend. Your personal physician will have medical coverage at all times for his or her patients if he or she is conscientious (this is a good question to ask on the first visit).

Frequency of Medical Visits

How often during a man's life does a physician need to be seen, presuming generally good health? The answer to this has become complicated by medical economics, so I shall simply present the ideal. This must be modified, obviously, by the reality of "managed care."

The years between ages eighteen and thirty-five are the healthiest of a man's life. A thorough physical examination, mostly for "baseline" purposes and to establish a medical relationship with the physician, should be done early on in this period. Assuming no problems are encountered routine medical visits, mainly for brief checkups, are advisable only every three to four years. If special problems are encountered, of course, special attention and follow-up visits are necessitated. The doctor will advise you on this frequency. If necessary, your primary physician may refer you to a specialist. This, incidentally, is preferable by far than going to see one on your own. For one thing, it is important for your personal doctor to know all that goes on with you medically; otherwise, mistakes in medication are easily made. Then, also, your specialist will have to be responsive and responsible to your personal doctor; a bit of important insurance. Types of specialists you may see during your medical life will, of course, depend upon your state of health and specific needs that may occur. For instance, appendicitis or a hernia calls for a surgeon. Eye examinations after the age of forty are best performed by an ophthalmologist (an M.D.), but may be quite satisfactorily done by an optometrist (non-M.D./O.D.). Ask your doctor. "Managed care" requires referral by your "gatekeeper" personal doctor, so you may have no choice in the matter, if you don't want to be responsible for an unpaid specialist's bill.

From the ages of thirty-five to fifty the visits, again presuming no obvious problems, should happen every two to three years, but the examinations will be more complex and inclusive in nature. Cancer detection becomes a concern in this period and special tests are in order (see "The Physical Examination").

From the age of fifty onward, yearly checkups are in order. The incidence and detection of preventable disease begins to accelerate and increases with age.

These general rules do not apply, of course, when there are special circumstances such as early-onset and asymptomatic disease such as hypertension or where family history of a disease such as diabetes or colon cancer, may increase the odds of particular ailments. And, of course, there are the "worried well." Some individuals just cannot rest without the reassurance of frequent periodic examination. If they can afford this luxury, why not? As long as the physician is aware of this mind-set the patient may, by such examination, prevent needless worry and overtreatment by overzealous practitioners who may prey upon this type of patient.

Alternative Medicine

Since the dawn of mankind, the search for wellness and immortality has spawned great stories and many directions. The branches that spring from the tree have been and still are many. These are the alternatives to conventional allopathy.

The National Institutes of Health (NIH) recently divided alternative medicine into seven treatment categories: 1) mind-body (biofeedback, meditation, yoga); 2) alternative medical practice (homeopathy, acupuncture); 3) diet and nutrition (macrobiotics, supplements); 4) "bioelectric" (electroacupuncture); 5) manual healing (touch, chiropractic, massage therapy); 6) herbal medicines (Asian, Latin American, Amerind); and 7) unproven pharmacologic methods (for example, shark cartilage, chelation therapy). Many of these methods are being studied at universities and the NIH itself, and the NIH Office of Alternative Medicine plans to publicize the results as they become available. It is estimated that as many as 40 percent of people avail themselves of these treatments at a considerable cost, about $14 billion in 1990, with most of it nonreimbursable by insurance. The majority of patients who are taking this alternative way, unfortunately, do not, for one reason or another, inform their physicians and this is too bad, if not downright dangerous. Many of these treatments have side effects that can cause problems or toxic reactions which, if kept from the doctor, may go unrecognized and untreated. It is important also for the physician to be knowledgeable about alternative medicine. Some of these alternative medical practices are of particular interest.

Naturopathy ("nature's path"). This is probably the oldest of the alternative healing disciplines, deriving from the ancient Egyptian cult of "wchtu." This system depended upon the observation of birds and animals along the Nile and led to the first notion of autointoxication. It was noticed, for instance, that animals were constantly defecating without regard to time or place, unlike civilized mankind that usually deferred this function to convenience. The Egyptians also noted that the sacred ibis bird (the god Thoth) would stand by the riverbank, dip its long beak into the sacred waters, and seemingly then give itself an enema! Actually the bird was rubbing its oil gland, which is adjacent to its anal opening, in order to preen and anoint its feathers. The Egyptians also noted that mummies did not deteriorate if the viscera were removed before mummification (bacteria of the gastrointestinal tract would not corrupt the body if removed and placed in separate burial jars). Ergo—disease could be prevented and treated by the use of a high-fiber diet, strong laxatives, and frequent enemas. This thinking has persisted to this day. Dr. John Harvey Kellogg of Battlecreek, Michigan, for instance, created a fabulously successful business and clinic that used these practices. There are many present-day practitioners of naturopathy and colonic therapy. There may actually be some basis for this wild-sounding idea. It seems that high-fiber diets and rapid transit through the gastrointestinal tract *is* beneficial. Cholesterol levels are lowered and bacterial conversion of certain foods, especially fats, to potentially cancer-stimulating substances, are curtailed. Dr. Denis

Burkitt theorized that the reason for the low incidence of cancer of the colon in black Africa is the high-vegetable-fiber, low-fat diet, plus frequent unrestricted elimination practices. Naturopathic theory, therefore, is not completely absurd. It may even be beneficial if not totally depended upon for a panacea. The diets have merit. One caveat, however: "Colon therapy," laxatives, and enemas, can be overdone and addicting. The normal bowel function may become overridden and laxatives and enemas may be required for normal elimination. Also, a few cases of disease transmission, particularly hepatitis and amebic dysentery from contaminated equipment, have been recorded. The naturopaths also advocate sunlight therapy, which is not advisable considering the adverse effects of ultraviolet rays on the skin and eyes (skin cancer and cataract formation).

Chiropractic. This is a system of therapy invented by Dr. Daniel Palmer in the late nineteenth century (1895–1898). He considered disease to be a result of pressure on spinal nerves by vertebrae that were dislocated or "subluxated." He theorized that manual manipulation of the spine and extremities would correct these deformities and cure disease.

Prior to this, in the mid-1800s, the osteopaths held similar notions but gradually they became convinced of the importance of conventional medical practices. For the most part, osteopaths have become allopathic physicians with some emphasis on physical medicine techniques (massage, gentle manipulation, and so on). Chiropractors, however, as a group, persist in Palmer's theory of causation of disease. They are not licensed to prescribe drugs or do surgery and, in my experience, no matter how erroneous some think their premise may be, many patients seem to benefit from chiropractic ministrations. I feel that such benefit may derive from the time spent talking to the patient as well as the soothing and beneficial effects of physical therapy and massage. One important warning: neck manipulation should be avoided! Serious spinal cord damage and even death have resulted from this, and the wisest chiropractors will avoid such potentially dangerous treatment. They will also refer patients to appropriate allopathic care if a serious disease seems to be present.

Homeopathy. Samuel Hahnemann (1775–1843) was a German physician who founded homeopathy on the theory that drugs produce symptoms in healthy people that mimic the symptoms that they relieve in the sick. Furthermore, he believed that minute doses of a drug will cure the disease that large doses of that drug will cause. This convolution was not entirely irrational, since the drugs used then were frequently deadly poisons, and by withdrawing them, cures were effected more often than not. Most disease, in otherwise healthy people, will subside naturally. In any case, the many schools of homeopathy were gradually absorbed into the allopathic schools, particularly after the Flexner Report and the rise of scientific medicine, but homeopathic practitioners and products have come roaring back in popularity in recent years. It does not seem at all likely that dilutions of medications to billionths parts (0 to 1 molecule of medicine per dose) can be at all effective, but it is so claimed. Again, if it seems to help, there is no harm as long as the treatment does not interfere with detection and management of serious disease.

Acupuncture. This refers to the ancient practice of Chinese medicine which purports to treat pain and disease by needle insertion into key spots mapped out on the body. The needle stimulation may be augmented by "moxibustion" or the burning of the herb "moxa" on the end of the inserted needle. A modern variation is electrical stimulation rather than fire. Supposedly these are "channels" (anatomically unknown) which convey the stimulating "fluid" to the place of trouble. For instance, a needle in the earlobe is said to help the addicted smoker or overeater. A physician friend of mine, while traveling in China, met an acupuncturist physician at an agricultural commune near Xian. When asked for a demonstration, the doctor inserted a long needle into the web of my friend's thumb which caused him to jump several feet into the air while screaming, "What's this for?" "Headache," was the reply. "You got a headache?" "No," said my friend. "See," said the doctor.

Acupuncture seems to work, at least for a while, for some painful conditions. The mechanisms are unknown but some evidence exists for stimulation of brain neurons to produce natural central nervous system painkillers, endorphins, by the acupuncture process via the peripheral nerve circuits. Apparently this effect may be strong enough to produce anesthesia for major surgery; however, it has not been used in the United States as far as I know. And as much as I looked for it in my medical tour of China, I personally saw no surgery using this form of anesthetic. I have never seen any serious systemic disease cured by acupuncture and no such cure has ever been documented, to my knowledge. If the process works in intolerable pain situations, I encourage its trial if I have nothing more effective to offer.

Holistic medicine. This bases itself on the concept of the "whole" person, as one's whole mind, body, spirit, and emotions are in balance with the environment. The holistic approach may include conventional and alternative methods of diagnosis and treatment including acupuncture, faith healing, body imagery, massage, megavitamin and herbal therapy, folk medicine, diet, meditation, and yoga. Surgery and prescription drugs are to be avoided and self-regulation of lifestyles toward healthy habits emphasized. Who can argue with this? A good allopathic physician will certainly subscribe to this philosophy—Hippocrates' third rule, Rx (or "regimen") meant coming to terms with one's environment in beneficial ways.

I have mentioned the possible and overt beneficial effects of these alternative modes of treatment. Allopathy, conventional medicine, is eclectic in thought and action. That is, the best and most useful modes of any and all of the branches of the healing tree, from high-fiber diets to spiritual healing, are part and parcel of my profession. We reject nothing that may help our patients. We do not slavishly go out on a limb of one of the branches, as seems to be the case with some of the alternative ways. Unfortunately, patients with otherwise incurable or terminal illness may lose hope and become vulnerable targets for those unscrupulous enough to prey upon them. This is particularly sad if we, the primary physicians, do not understand and deal sympathetically and adequately with their pain. Here, certain of the alternatives are of real and particular help; for example, mental imagery in cancer therapy, biofeedback and acupuncture in pain management, or music therapy for depressed or demented patients.

Herbal and natural remedies. I have already referred to the use of these non-proven substances, some of which are now in common use. A few of these materials (e.g., St. John's wort, Ginkgo biloba, ginseng, zinc lozenges, creatine, garlic, echinacea, etc.) may indeed have some beneficial effects worthy of further (controlled and scientific) study, and indeed some are now being legitimately investigated. In the meanwhile, a billion dollar industry has sprung up by virtue of the uncontrolled sales of these "nutropharmaceuticals" as food supplements, not only by health-food stores but now also by some drug companies eager to get in on the profits. The FDA cannot regulate this industry since the producers of these supplements are careful not to claim a medical effect; they simply imply such, not having to prove anything. Standards of purity and dosage are not controlled and it would appear that little governmental effort to protect the public is pending.

DR. DASHE'S TIPS FOR HEALTH MAINTENANCE

1. Having a physician who knows you and is someone you're comfortable with is important; if you haven't got one, take steps to get one today.

2. Know the constraints your health plan has on your decision-making process; contact your agent or company representative about your needs and concerns.

3. Ask your friends and colleagues for referrals, keeping in mind the type of doctor you can relate to, and check the doctor's credentials.

4. Don't wait for a physical problem to go see the doctor, make an appointment while you're healthy and save yourself surprises later on.

5. Interview your doctor, get some further information on credentials and other background information, and get an idea of the overall style of the doctor. Ask questions!

6. Arrange to have an initial history and physical exam performed so the doctor is prepared when a visit becomes a necessity.

7. Keep a copy of all your records somewhere safe at home, including information on various illnesses, family history, allergies, and immunizations.

8. The older you get the more often you'll need to get an examination. Early detection of certain diseases could save your life.

9. Ask as many questions as you need to in order to feel informed. I hope you will have found a doctor who is willing to give you answers that will satisfy your curiousity and let you play an active role in your treatment.

10. If you choose an alternative medicine practitioner, make sure you know what you are going to get at what price, and understand the possible risks as well as the possible benefits.

Chapter 3

THE PHYSICAL EXAMINATION

I hadn't seen Dr. Martin Stone (name changed for obvious reasons), a man in his forties, for at least ten years. He had once been my intern at UCLA and had become a successful and well-regarded ophthalmologist. He came to my office for an annual physical examination, which had been his routine. He had decided to change physicians because his previous doctor seemed to be unimpressed with his complaint that he was no longer able to swim fifty laps in his pool on the weekend; he was down to thirty-five laps. He had no other complaints at this time except for perhaps a slight increase of fatiguability lately. He had always been healthy. He was annoyed with his doctor's attitude, which he ascribed to the frequent and ironic lack of attention some doctors provide to physician-patients.

Well, Martin looked "funny" to me. He was definitely paler and sallower than I remembered him to be and he seemed rather tired. I questioned and examined him methodically, as I would any new patient; a habit learned from bitter experience—assume nothing. My friend had all the hallmarks of severe anemia. Pallor, sallowness, and loss of pinkness of his mucus membranes. He looked sick but he didn't feel sick. This usually means that the anemia, which means loss of blood hemoglobin, the red stuff that carries oxygen to our tissues, was of gradual onset, over a period of months. Since men don't menstruate, blood loss, the most frequent cause of anemia, must be from the bowel. But he had no history of visible blood loss from "either end" and I had done a rectal examination which showed no evidence of occult (hidden) seepage. My colleague was, therefore, suffering from some form of major chronic anemia, something bad such as leukemia perhaps. I shuddered at the thought as I asked him again, reviewing his history, was he sure that he or any member of his family did not have a history of severe anemia? He thought again. He had forgotten his mother, he vaguely recalled, had once told him that she had been diagnosed with pernicious anemia. That was it! Of all the blood disorders he could have had, this was by far the best. Appropriate laboratory studies were done in the next few days and the diagnosis of pernicious anemia confirmed. He was profoundly anemic with only 20 percent of the normal hemoglobin level! He was given the first of the periodic injections of vitamin B12 that he would require for the rest of his life. He felt better immediately and within a few weeks he was his usual predisease vigorous and athletic self. Pernicious anemia is a vitamin B12 deficiency disease, frequently inherited, caused by the inability of the gastrointestinal tract to absorb this vital substance. Before the discovery of this process and its treatment, it was invariably fatal. Now it is easily and totally curable. It is one of the truly great achievements of modern medical science, but it would have done nothing for Dr. Martin Stone had he not come in for his routine physical examination.

Once your doctor has been chosen, a basic history and physical examination is warranted. I will briefly outline what this is and why each step is important.

History

First of all comes a thorough medical history. This is by far the most important part of the examination. I have learned and taught over the years that careful listening is the most fruitful part of the doctor-patient relationship. The presence and diagnosis of disease (or health) is best discerned here. Sherlock Holmes, that fabulous diagnostician, was formulated by Sir Arthur Conan Doyle (a physician) from his observations of his professor of medicine, Dr. Bell, at work. By carefully listening to and observing a person, one can obtain an enormous body of knowledge about that individual. The physician will ask how the patient feels now. The past history of previous illnesses or operations will be reviewed. The family history, particularly regarding immediate family (mother, father, siblings, aunts, uncles, grandparents), may give clues to family disease traits, genetic and otherwise (particular exposures, diet, and so on). Current habits, especially the use of tobacco, alcohol, and medicines are discussed, as are allergies to foods or drugs. An accurate history of previous immunizations and vaccinations is taken.

Review of Systems

The physician will discuss the various systems in detail and ask about symptoms. For example:

Skin: rashes and sensitivities;

Lymph nodes: swollen glands;

Head: headaches;

Eyes: vision, glasses, blurring, blackouts;

Ears: changes in hearing, drainage, pain;

Nose: congestion, bleeding;

Mouth: dental problems, difficulty chewing or swallowing;

Cardiorespiratory: shortness of breath, chest discomfort, palpitations;

Gastrointestinal: Recurrent nausea, vomiting, diarrhea, constipation, bowel habits, blood in the stools, jaundice, or liver history;

Genitourinary: venereal disease, pain or problems with urinating, bloody or odd-colored urine, sexual problems, premature ejaculation, impotency, rashes or warts on the penis, sexual preferences or practices;

Neuromuscular: Weakness or paralysis, pain or limitation of muscles, sensation disturbances (numbness, tingling, pain);

Bones and joints: arthritis or rheumatism, swelling, limitations of motion, backache, neckache;

Neuropsychologic: Fainting, convulsions, memory loss, delusions, hallucinations, depression, obsessions, compulsions.

After all these systems are explored, the doctor again will ask if any additional information has been remembered. It's a good idea for the prepared patient to have these historical items listed, either on paper or mentally. It helps and it saves everybody's time. Currently, it is not uncommon for a nurse or paramedical person to take the history, but at the least the doctor should carefully review it.

Physical Examination

The actual physical examination is next. Much of it has already been done; your physician has already observed a great deal about you. Your mood, your nutritional status, your appearance of health or not, your youthfulness (or not), your intelligence, your ability to cope with the stress of the examination, your apparent emotional state. The physician is trained to observe these things and to put them into context. The actual "hands on" exam is next.

A careful physical examination should be thorough and reasonably swift. The patient should be asked to undress. Modesty is preserved by appropriate "cover-ups." Men are usually permitted to keep on their briefs until the final examination of the urogenital region.

The vital signs (pulse rate, respiratory rate, temperature, and blood pressure), and the patient's height and weight usually will have been taken and recorded by the nursing aides but may be rechecked by the doctor if any abnormality is noted. The general appearance, nutritional state, and fitness is noted. A systematic examination is then carried out as follows:

Skin: Texture, color, hair distribution, and pigmentation are noted.

Lymph nodes: All groups (neck, armpits, groin especially) are palpated (examined by touch and feel).

Head: Notes are made regarding the shape of the skull and hair distribution.

Eyes: The pupils' reactivity to light, eye motions, visual acuity, the lens, and retina are examined using an ophthalmoscope. The retina is the only place that arteries and veins can be seen directly without surgery. Textbooks have been written about the many systemic diseases that can be diagnosed by an eye examination, from arteriosclerosis to zoster (shingles).

Ears: Hearing is tested with a tuning fork. (I also use my watch tick.) Shape and size of the external ears are noted; they may give clues to systemic disease. For instance, low-set ears may signify congenital kidney disease; coronary artery disease may be associated with deep creases in the ear lobes. The ear canals and the ear drums are examined with the aid of a lighted instrument known as an otoscope, which is inserted gently into the ear canal. (Patients usually ask if I can see through to the other side. Heh, heh.)

Nose: Nasal passages are checked for congestion, bleeding, deviation of the septum. (Most people have a deviated septum and it's usually of no significance.)

Mouth: It is very important to look thoroughly at the tongue and mucus membranes. Early changes that may be precancerous may be detected and treated. The teeth and gums are inspected, not only for presence of dental disease, which is important enough, but the state of the teeth also may mirror systemic disease. For example, gum pigmentation may be seen with lead poisoning; a wide spacing of the teeth may be associated with a tumor of the pituitary gland. The back of the throat, the tonsils, the uvula (that funny little piece of flesh that hangs back there) may all have stories to tell the trained observer.

Thorax (chest): Symmetry and shape are noted. A wide front-to-back dimension may mean lung disease. Movement should be even and not strained. Excess breast tissue in a man is embarrassing and abnormal, and may indicate disease; therefore, the breasts are examined.

Lungs: Tapping of the chest (percussion) determines the position and size of the heart, lungs, diaphragm, dome of the liver, and other abdominal organs (viscera). It also may determine if abnormal fluid is present. Listening to the chest (auscultation) with a stethoscope permits detection of abnormal breathing sounds, and the heart sounds, rhythm, and valve function are noted.

Peripheral vessels: The veins are examined for varicosity (bulging due to valve failure). The pulses in the extremities are felt in order to see whether the blood supply is adequate and equal and whether arteriosclerotic changes (such as hardening) are occurring in the arteries.

Abdomen: Examination includes feeling for the normal organ placement and size, especially the liver, spleen, and large bowel. Occasionally the kidneys can be felt and, if full, the bladder. The doctor searches for abnormal masses in the abdomen and uses the stethoscope again to listen for the bowel sounds. Atypical pulses or murmurs, such as may be present with blood vessel abnormalities, are noted if present.

Genitalia: The penis, scrotum, and testicles are carefully palpated. Of special importance is the scrotum, where lumps and bumps can represent early tumors. The inguinal (groin) areas are examined for hernias. The doctor inserts the tip of the small finger into the base of the scrotum on both sides and asks for the famous "cough please." He will feel a hernia as a lump coming down to meet the fingertip with this maneuver.

Back and extremities: The posture and mobility of the spine will be examined next, and then the motion and appearance of the movable joints. Loss of motion, deformity, swelling (edema), and inflammation (arthritis) are excluded or noted.

Neurological system: The reflexes are tested by tapping the tendons with a rubber hammer. Surprisingly, all of our muscles have reflexes and all can be so tested. The reflexes should be present in the majority of muscles tested and be symmetrical and not too active. Overactivity may be just as abnormal as underactivity. (Incidentally, reflex activity has nothing to do with sanity.) The strength of the muscles, too, are tested and should be symmetrical and adequate to perform usual daily functions such as standing, grasping, pulling, and so on. Sensory examination includes touching, pain (via a pinprick), heat perception, and special senses such as spatial position and balance. For instance, you may be asked to touch the tip of your nose with the tip of an index finger with your eyes closed. Or you may be asked to stand on one foot with your eyes closed.

Last but not least is the *dreaded rectal examination*. It's not so bad; look what women have to go through. I shall never forget the day that our esteemed, dignified, and well-loved professor of physical diagnosis at the University of California San Francisco Medical School, Dr. Leroy Briggs, announced solemnly to us downy-faced sophomore medical students, "Everyone has a rectum. Put your finger in it. If you don't, you'll put your foot in it." He then ordered that forthwith we would practice this on one another before we would be let loose on patients. It was, I recall, a humiliating, humbling, and interesting experience, worse than learning to ride a bike, but not as painful. Remember, then, we all had to go through it, doctors not excepted. A good thing, too. One medical school, in its wise decision to let medical students learn how it feels to be a patient, requires that all male students be placed up in stirrups, legs apart, at which point a strange female doctor enters the room, squeezes the subject's testicles, mutters something dire and unintelligible, and exits without further discussion or questioning.

Anyway, Briggs was correct. Many a life has been saved by this brief experience. Cancers of the prostate and rectum are major killers of men and the rectal examination is an important method of detection. Of course, the incidence of these and the other serious detectable diseases in the asymptomatic man is age related. So, usually, the routine examination is not urged until the age of thirty-five unless there are reasons (symptoms or family history). Truly, it is a swift and not especially painful examination. A tip to the examinee: strain down against the offending finger. This actually relaxes the anal sphincter, spasm of which is the main cause of physical discomfort. The mental anguish goes away rapidly, too. The procedure consists of an external examination, where the physician

Figure 3-1: CONDUCTING THE DIGITAL RECTAL EXAMINATION

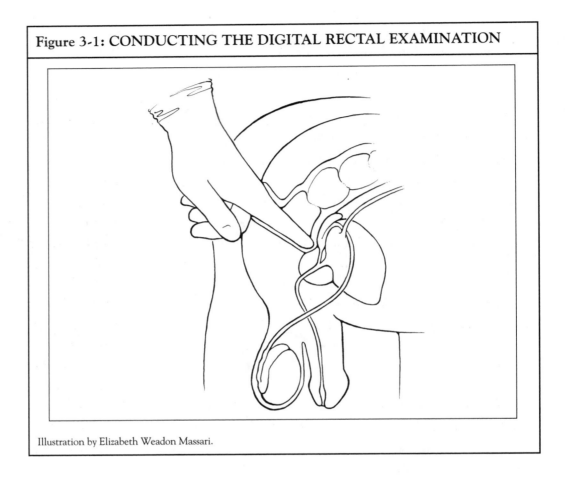

Illustration by Elizabeth Weadon Massari.

looks for hemorrhoids ("piles" or varicose veins of the anus and rectum), warts, and other skin abnormalities. The lubricated, gloved finger is gently introduced and the ano-rectal structures palpated. Abnormal masses are easily felt. The prostate gland is directly palpable below the finger (Figure 3-1) and its size, shape, and consistency are important traits to be noted. Asymmetry, undue tenderness, enlargement, or nodules may denote diseases that require further investigation and treatment. The stool residue on the glove is then tested chemically for the presence of blood or pus, indicators of colon problems.

I cannot emphasize strongly enough the importance of this procedure (although I always give my patients the option of skipping it, if fear of it will keep a man away from the doctor and *any* kind of examination).

Laboratory Tests

I was taught, and still believe, that the face-to-face history and thorough examination is the most important part of the practice of medicine. It is not only diagnostic, but is unquestionably therapeutic. The patient always feels better afterward, having been given the hands-on evidence of a caring physician's interest. Even if no medicines are prescribed and no surgical manipulation performed, anxiety is relieved and healing begins. (This is the "alternative medicine" that most people seek, I believe.) It is a mixed blessing, therefore, that the past fifty years have given us truly remarkable diagnostic laboratory procedures which have made diagnosis and treatment simpler, faster, and more reliable. I can't imagine, for instance, how we were able to manage without a CAT or MRI scan, or chemistry or blood autoanalyzers. But manage we did, as best we could. While I am in no way ready to give up these marvelous tools, I must point out that they are, for the most part, confirmatory to the diagnostic notions formed by the history and physical examination. There is not yet an electronic physician that will accept a patient into its test chamber, process him, and deliver him from illness, cured and content. Nice idea, but still some way off! The downside of the laboratory revolution is the fact that medical schools and doctors have become too dependent on laboratory testing and may be, I fear, neglecting the basics. Not only is this unwise and costly, but it is dehumanizing and, in my view, bad medicine. I will describe some of these useful laboratory procedures.

Routine Laboratory Procedures

As part of a routine physical examination, a few tests should be performed, the routineness depends upon the age of the patient and his stage of life. For instance:

1. Urinalysis is useful in all instances. The presence of abnormal substances such as sugar, protein, blood, and so on, may indicate an unforeseen ailment. It is a rapid test, done with a "dipstick" and

occasionally microscopically, if warranted. It is a simple, useful gauge of kidney function and potential disease, and also serves as a screening tool for tumors and infections of the genitourinary tract (kidney, ureters, bladder, and urethra). This test should be performed routinely in men of all ages.

2. Complete blood count. This too should be a routine test for examinees of all ages. It is a simple measurement of the major components of the blood (hemoglobin, red and white cells, and so on), done rapidly these days by a wonderful, complex machine. A blood sample is fed into the machine and in a matter of a minute or two out pops a printout of all the necessary information. If any abnormalities are detected, microscopic examination of the blood may be done by a technician or hematologist. Anemias and a long list of disorders are thus diagnosable.

3. Blood chemistries. A truly amazing sight to see is a blood chemistry autoanalyzer. These robotic devices can do in a matter of minutes, or at most hours, with greater accuracy, what used to take hordes of technicians days and weeks. Even with automation, however, there are more technicians than ever. This is the result of the increase in availability of laboratory studies and the consequent greater use of them. The cost of a "panel" of the blood assays, from seven to twenty-five or so tests from one small blood specimen, is less than the cost of one or two tests of years ago. An example of such a panel is seen in Figure 3-2. These tests include such important information as liver and kidney function and different substances in the blood.

In addition to giving information about current problems, some of these tests may inform us of potential problems. For example, the cholesterol figures may warn of increased risk of later cardiovascular disease. One interesting outcome of these cheap and easily performed laboratory panels is the discovery that many normal and asymptomatic individuals have abnormal tests, which may indicate that some previously considered rare diseases are more common and benign than ever believed. The best example of this paradox is the serum calcium test that shows a slight elevation in many apparently

Figure 3-2: TYPICAL CHEMISTRY PANEL	
TEST	**MEASURES**
GLUCOSE	BLOOD SUGAR
TOTAL PROTEIN	BLOOD PROTEINS
ALBUMIN	
GLOBULIN	
SGOT	LIVER FUNCTION
SGPT	
ALKALINE PHOSPHATASE	
BILIRUBIN	
LDH	
URIC ACID	CHEMICAL INVOLVED IN GOUT
BLOOD UREA NITROGEN	KIDNEY FUNCTION
CREATININE	
PHOSPHOROUS	
SODIUM	MAJOR BLOOD MINERALS AND SALTS
POTASSIUM	
CALCIUM	
CHLORIDES	
CHOLESTEROL (TOTAL)	BLOOD FATS
TRIGLYCERIDES	
HDL, LDL, CHOLESTEROL	"GOOD" AND "BAD" CHOLESTEROL

healthy people. The cause, parathyroid gland overactivity, is a lot more frequent than ever suspected and, it seems, may not cause trouble enough to warrant anything more than observation over the years. At least, however, your physician has been alerted to this possibility and will know what to look for in future examinations. It would seem wise and prudent to have such a chemistry panel test done as a routine baseline early on, for example in the second or third decade at least and then whenever a general examination is performed again. It is cheap enough now to be cost effective and invaluable in preventive medicine.

One word about thyroid function tests. They have become precise and indicative of thyroid over- or underactivity and they, too, are relatively inexpensive and, in perspective, cost effective. A thyroid screening chemistry test costs about $20. Former President Bush had a yearly thorough comprehensive examination at Bethesda Naval Hospital that required, because he was president, two days of hospitalization and probably six figures' worth of sophisticated testing, but no thyroid screening test. This hospitalization, which no current insurance company would approve for any of us commoners, was followed by Mr. Bush's excursion into "Desert Storm," which then was closely followed by his development of a heart arrhythmia (a rapid, irregular heartbeat) and obvious mental and physical signs of thyroid overactivity. The man had been suffering from hyperthyroidism, probably for at least a year when looked at in retrospect. When asked why the diagnosis was missed, the president's staff of physician-professors responded that thyroid screening tests (all $20 or $30 worth) are not cost effective. I believe that thyroid screening is cost effective. Others can debate the cost effectiveness of Desert Storm.

4. Chest x-ray. This simple study is useful as a baseline for the first general adult examination. It conveys information about lungs and heart (shape, size, configuration) as well as the thoracic spine and bones. It need not be a routine, yearly event unless there is a special indication such as preexisting disease or symptoms such as a chronic

cough. Smokers, or people at special industrial risk (miners, chemical workers) need to have routine chest x-rays at one-to-three-year intervals.

5. Electrocardiogram (ECG or EKG). A resting electrocardiographic tracing of the heart used to be a basic test in the annual general physical examination, particularly for the male when heart concerns were thought to be primarily a masculine problem. Of course we know now that heart disease is a unisex problem. The cardiogram currently is seen to be a quaint custom, of little value to men or women, considering all the new things available. I refer to stress tests (treadmill) with and without nuclear or ultrasound (echocardiogram) addition. These studies are far more valuable and precise as diagnostic tools of heart disease, but they cannot be considered routine in all except the most financially devil-may-care instances. A simple treadmill ECG currently costs in the range of $400 to $600. This test, I believe, should be done only when there is a good reason; for example, symptoms, special risk factors, strong family history. A resting ECG, much less expensive, may be useful again as a baseline study, perhaps for later comparison but not necessarily a routine part of the general physical examination.

6. Special tests. It is important, when discussing laboratory studies, to understand the two major types of examinations that have changed medical practice for all time. These are the CAT or CT (computerized axial tomography) x-ray scan and the MRI (magnetic resonance imaging) scan. These studies, barely thirty years old, have given us the ability to visualize our insides as never before, without subjecting us to surgery. Gone is much of the guesswork and the exploratory surgeries. We can have three-dimensional anatomic views of our living bodies, any part and without dissection. The CT depends upon a computer analysis of multiple x-ray pictures. The MRI, which uses no x-ray irradiation, remarkably measures and puts into visual form our soft tissues and liquids (blood) and bone, by harmlessly "spinning" our very atoms with a strong magnet. Who, indeed, would have thought it possible? These miracles are by no means part of

routine laboratory examinations but most of us, sometime or other, will probably benefit from their existence.

7. Prostatic specific antigen (PSA). There is controversy whether this test, used for early detection of cancer of the prostate, should be routine. It has become so in many places, at least for men over forty years of age. I shall discuss this test in a later section (see "Genitourinary").

Adult Immunizations

A very important part of the routine examination is a review of vaccinations and immunizations. This is the best time, also, to take whatever boosters, or if warranted, primary immunizations. There are new vaccines, such as varicella-zoster (chickenpox) and hepatitis A, available, and newer ones yet in development. Indications for immunizations are changing, too, particularly because of the resurgence of antibiotic-resistant disease. I have, for example, urged all my adult patients to take Pneumococcal pneumonia vaccination because of the emergence of resistant strains of the previously easily killed bacteria. Health authorities consider this vaccine mandatory only for those over age sixty-four or at special risk. I disagree with this policy. I see no reason, cost effectiveness included, to give up the window of opportunity for prevention. Similarly influenza, though not currently a deadly disease, is nasty enough to warrant protection in all adults, and not just the elderly. Measles, mumps, rubella (German measles), and now chickenpox, are so-called childhood diseases, but are by no means innocuous for unprotected adults. Most Americans have either had the immunization during childhood or, in the case of chickenpox, the disease. If not, immunization is not only warranted, but may be critical. Even whooping cough (pertussis), thought to be limited to children, has recently been found to be a cause of many cases of persistent adult bronchitis and cough. Booster doses of a new fluid pertussis vaccine for adults may become routine soon. Polio seems to have been almost totally eliminated from the Western world through vaccination. The Sabin or oral vaccine, when given to one person, frequently immunized a whole family via its live viral transmission. Polio vaccination still must be kept up since the disease exists in many parts of the world, and it doesn't take long for a population to lose its immunity when vaccination stops. The only infectious disease of mankind that appears to have been totally eradicated is smallpox. The World Health Organization systematically chased this plague to the farthest corners of the earth, and by vaccinating everyone at risk, gave us a smallpox-free world. But the cost of stopping routine smallpox vaccination of the world's population is that there is no longer resistance to this disease. If the virus were to reappear, a large portion of humanity would die, as in the plagues of the Middle Ages, until a resistant population again emerged.

We would very much like to totally eliminate such diseases as polio and hepatitis as we were able to do with smallpox. Efforts continue but so far, for socioeconomic reasons and others, it seems unlikely to happen. It thus, behooves us, the lucky ones, to see to it that we and our children are protected and stay protected. For example:

1. Diphtheria-tetanus. This adult vaccine should be given to every adult who missed the childhood vaccine. A booster is needed every ten years, or sooner if a particularly dirty wound is present.
2. Measles, mumps, rubella. Again, for those not infected or vaccinated as a child, especially those born after 1956, vaccination is necessary.
3. Influenza. This vaccine should be taken yearly because new strains appear. This is especially important for those over sixty.
4. Pneumonia vaccine. All adults, especially the elderly and those at particular risk (those with chronic disease), should have this vaccine. This is a long-lasting vaccine and the time for boosters has not been determined; at a minimum every six years, perhaps much longer.
5. Hepatitis B. Children are now being vaccinated routinely against hepatitis B. Adults, if immunity is not present on blood testing, should receive this vaccination. People at special risk are health workers, housemates of infected people, IV drug users, or anyone with multiple sex partners.

6. Hepatitis A. This is the epidemic food-borne type of hepatitis. I recommend this vaccine, particularly to travelers to unsanitary places (much of the world).

7. Chickenpox. This is a new vaccine advisable for anyone who hasn't had the disease.

8. Special vaccinations for travelers to exotic lands. Check with your physician or local health department. Such vaccines as yellow fever, meningitis, plague, typhoid (oral, or a new injectable kind if one is in a hurry), cholera, and encephalitis may be advisable. They are not routine in this country.

9. Malaria. At this time, there is no vaccine for malaria, probably still the most prominent and deadly of the tropical diseases. Prophylaxis with various antimalarial drugs (for example, Lariam®, Chloroquine®, quinine, doxycycline) will vary with the country of destination. Again, check with your doctor or local public health authority.

In summary then, your routine examination may, if you are fortunate, do nothing more than reassure you that you are hale and hearty, which news should put a little additional spring in your step. On the other hand, it may save your life or prevent serious illness and disability, as it did for my young colleague Dr. Stone. In any case, it may pick up evidence of avoidable future problems. Preventive medicine is far preferable to *ER* or *Chicago Hope*. One needs to have immunizations reviewed and brought up to date, and baseline medical measurements are vital and valuable for the future.

Men are seemingly reluctant to see the doctor at all, much less to have physical examinations. This attitude is clearly shortsighted, particularly since so much can be achieved. So, swallow your stubbornness, your denial of your own mortality, your machismo, and turn yourself in, before someone else does. Sometimes, too, you may need a doctor, so it's nice to have one to call.

DR. DASHE'S TIPS FOR HEALTH MAINTENANCE

1. If you haven't had an exam in a while (and the older you get, "a while" can get shorter) or you've changed doctors, schedule an examination.

2. If you are hesitating to make that appointment, you are not alone. Many men hate to have exams for a variety of ill-founded reasons. Don't let your fear, trepidation, modesty, or machismo intervene in your health care concerns.

3. Shrugging and grunting is a poor way of communicating. Make sure that you give your doctor a complete and thorough medical history, and answer questions honestly and completely. Come prepared with your medical history in hand.

4. The physical part of the exam can seem intrusive and occasionally embarrassing. Try asking questions about each part of the physical exam; it's good to know what's going on.

5. The dreaded and shunned rectal examination is extremely important and potentially life saving; furthermore, it ain't so bad!

6. Expect routine laboratory tests; the extent varying with age, history, and physical findings. It is not uncommon to have a urinalysis, complete blood count, blood chemistries, thyroid function, chest x-ray, and electrocardiogram.

7. Prostate problems and colon cancer are common to men, and testing in the area is becoming more routine. Once again, early detection can make all the difference in treatment.

8. Review, record, and keep your immunizations up-to-date; especially flu shots and pneumonia vaccine.

9. A reasonable schedule of future medical visits may be planned for you. If not, be sure to ask.

Chapter 4

WHEN TO CALL
A DOCTOR

The grxeat Stoic philosopher Seneca said, "Ignore pain, either it will go away or you will." This is probably the case. However, the endpoint may leave something to be desired, at least in some instances. Clearly, the ancient Greeks and Romans worried enough about health to warrant Seneca's remark, but there was little enough that could be done in those days to suggest anything else but resignation. This is no longer the case.

The healthy human is not totally immune to physical trouble. By far, most ailments are transient and (in retrospect) trivial. But how is one to tell? Experience helps, of course, but lacking this there are some guidelines to follow.

Pain

Sure, it hurts, but where? An ache in the back or in an extremity, while annoying and even momentarily incapacitating, is usually easily self-diagnosed (as either a sprain or strain) or treated with minor analgesics such as acetaminophen

(Tylenol®), aspirin, ibuprofen (Advil®), and so on. Rest, hot or cold compresses, and time usually are all that is necessary for resolution.

Occasional *headaches* are managed by these same simple measures.

Abdominal cramps are frequently accompanied by gas or diarrhea and respond to time, abstinence from eating, and simple medications, such as Imodium® or Pepto-Bismol®.

Heartburn usually responds to antacids. Duration and location of the pain is critical. If, despite simple measures, pain persists or worsens, medical advice is needed.

Chest pain, however, is another matter. People, particularly those over the age of thirty-five, must be concerned with the possibility of coronary artery disease. I would be terribly remiss in suggesting that chest pain, particularly that which is persistent (over one hour), severe, associated with sweating or nausea, or brought on by physical or emotional exertion, be ignored. Most of the time the problem is not heart disease, although this is the frequent subject of the anxious calls that doctors receive. (My own personal rule of thumb is, if anyone calls with the statement that "I'm having a heart attack," it hardly ever is. I worry about the guy who says, "Oh doc, I know it's nothing, but this thing in my chest and shoulder won't go away.") Denial seems to click into place when serious disease signals to a man. Heaven help him if, as so many poor victims have done, they try to "run it off!" If chest pain is severe and a doctor is not readily available for advice, a 911 call is justified. Paramedics are well equipped to save heart attack victims early on. Getting to an emergency room promptly is of paramount importance. The new clot-dissolving drugs and early intervention with angiography and angioplasty can not only save the patient now, but may add years to a person's life by preserving the cardiac muscle from destruction.

Fever

This symptom usually denotes inflammation or infection someplace in the body. A fever is defined as an elevation of body temperature. Body temperature is not a steady 98.6 degrees Fahrenheit (37.5 degrees Celsius). It varies from day to night and from person to person. A body temperature of less than 99.5 degrees oral (rectal is 1 degree higher normally) is of little concern. Usually a subnormal temperature is not of significance unless one is suffering from hypothermia or prolonged exposure to cold.

The presence of other localizing symptoms is of importance. If one has a runny nose, cough, and sore throat, upper respiratory infection is obvious. If painful urination or gastrointestinal symptoms are present, gastrointestinal or genitourinary infections are likely. In any case, if symptoms are vague or alarming or persist more than three days (for example, coughing up pus or blood or yellow nasal discharge), then medical advice is warranted.

Bleeding

A cut that bleeds profusely is a frightening symptom. However, if bleeding stops with simple pressure (with Kleenex®, sterile pad, or finger), the emergency ceases. This includes nosebleeds, which one can almost always stop by holding the nostrils firmly for five minutes (forget the ice cubes and the various positions which direct the blood down your throat). Persistent bleeding or bleeding from any other orifice needs medical attention. The rate determines the urgency. (A little blood goes a long way and a teaspoonful will color a toilet bowl like a Hawaiian sunset.) So call, but don't panic! It usually isn't cancer!

Trauma

Okay, it hurts. If you can move it, it probably isn't broken. Fractured limbs or spine usually will lay you low, will continue to hurt intensely, and you will know it and seek medical attention sooner or later. It is best not to try to move if fracture is suspected unless there is no other way to seek help. Head trauma, particularly involving unconsciousness, momentary or not, rates aid by a physician, or at least a phone call, and if unconsciousness persists, a 911 call.

Bite wounds, animal or human, require medical attention. They are always unclean. Insect and spider stings are no cause for alarm unless there is a history of allergies or the spider is brown or black. Topical hydrocortisone and oral antihistamines may be used to treat ordinary bites. Sometimes rubbing in a paste of meat tenderizer (Adolph's® mixed with water) will prevent allergic inflammation, if you're at home and it is handy.

Other

Upper respiratory infections. The ubiquitous "cold" (sneezing, sore throat followed frequently by cough within a day or so) is treated by grandma better than by medical science. You all know the drill: aspirin or acetaminophen, tea with honey and lemon, chicken soup. The misery, aching, and malaise will go away in three to four days. If, however, three days pass and you're worse, have a fever over 100 degrees F, have begun to snort or spit yellow mucus, it's a cold no longer and antibiotics may be helpful. Antibiotics do not cure colds. Indeed, it's unwise to treat colds and other viral infections with them. You may need them later and have, by too early use, made them ineffective for your particular bug.

Flu or influenza ("la grippe") is a different and interesting story. There is the tendency to call all gastrointestinal and upper respiratory infections "flu." They aren't and the distinction is important. True influenza is a specific viral disease with a deadly history. More people died of true influenza (some 25 million) during the pandemic (an epidemic involving the whole world) of 1917–1921 than all the previous plagues of mankind, including the Black Death of the fourteenth to sixteenth centuries. The flu virus has variations known as A and B, with slight geographical differences (for example, Hong Kong variety). The illness is characteristic and is definitely not a cold. True influenza is always accompanied by a dry, wracking cough and severe aching malaise. Fever, up to 103 degrees F is usual but only for three days. Recovery is usually dramatic, with the fourth day bringing an end to the aching, fever, and cough but leaving one feeling like the proverbial dishrag, maybe for a week or so. If fever, malaise, and other symptoms continue, such as coughing up pink or blood-streaked sputum, it isn't flu anymore. Pneumonia has probably jumped in. Call, if you haven't already done so. Most patients are, in my experience, alarmed enough by the initial symptoms of true flu and call early on. This is just as well since there are drugs which are effective in treating this virus; at least, they decrease the length and severity of symptoms. These medicines, amantadine (Symmetrel®) and rimanadine (Flumadine®) if given prior to symptoms (during an epidemic or after exposure to an infected person) can actually prevent the disease caused by flu virus-A strains. Better yet, flu immunizations are very effective and there is no reason why all adults should not take them. Currently, yearly boosters are necessary since the active flu strains vary from year to year. I, personally, have taken them every year and, despite much exposure, have been free of this nasty disease. In addition, pneumonia vaccination (as of now, one shot works indefinitely) is a marvelous but sadly underutilized vaccination. Resistant Pneumococcal pneumonia is a present future plague. Persistent respiratory symptoms such as cough, low-grade fever (99.5 degrees to 100.5 degrees), and funny-looking sputum, require medical intervention and, probably, a chest x-ray. Chronic nasal congestion or yellow mucus are also best handled by your doctor.

Gastrointestinal. Acute nausea and vomiting with or without diarrhea, "GI flu" is a common urban plague, frequently running wild through a family. You could die, you think, but you don't. The green-tinged skin sported by the victims of this viral gastroenteritis alarms all who view it. Also alarming is the tendency of the viree to faint when springing up to run to the toilet bowl. The major danger from this disease is the subsequent fall to the floor with the attendant bruising. Symptoms usually last no more than twenty-four vivid hours with miraculous, spontaneous recovery the rule. However, the extreme symptoms usually elicit a call to the doctor. An antinausea medicine, such as under-the-tongue Bucladin® or a rectal suppository (Compazine®, Vistaril®) may be prescribed and helpful. Imodium A-D and Pepto-Bismol are helpful for diarrhea, once vomiting has stopped. Most important is avoidance of eating during the acute stage. Little sips of water, soda, or tea will prevent serious dehydration. As for the rest of the gastrointestinal symptoms—pain, heartburn, diarrhea, blood—if any of these things are persistent or severe at onset, get on the phone!

Genitourinary. Unless it is a simple or transient symptom, such as a momentary discomfort while urinating, just about anything amiss with the plumbing department needs consultation with your doctor. This includes painful urination, frequency or urgency when urinating, discharge, blood, pain in the penis or testicles, rash, and most important, any swelling or lumpiness in or on the penis or the scrotum. These structures require hands-on maintenance. The scrotum and the testicles should be felt carefully during the shower. Sexual problems, such as premature ejaculation, impotency, and loss of libido (sexual desire) are also treatable and consultable conditions which we will deal with in a later section of this book.

Neurological. Symptoms of dizziness, weakness, numbness, inability to walk, talk, or use one's limbs or any alteration of consciousness or senses (sight, hearing, and so on) may be of serious consequence and require rapid medical consultation. Likewise serious or persistent emotional troubles. We'll discuss these later, too.

Self-Treatment

The old saw goes, "A doctor who treats himself has a fool for a physician." Now it can be added "maybe." I will reiterate: most illnesses, by far, clear up themselves within a few days. I have mentioned some situations that require medical help, occasionally right away. The situation is further complicated nowadays by the managed care system, which often comes between the patient and swift contact with his doctor. Also, more and more previously prescription only medicines are becoming available over the counter. This is a double-edged sword, I believe. Illnesses may be self-treated erroneously or inadequately. A few guidelines:

1. If you are sick and scared, call, for heaven's sake. This is no time for heroism!
2. If you are not getting better by three days, call!
3. If simple measures, such as aspirin, acetaminophen, antacids, Pepto-Bismol, chicken soup, and hot tea aren't helping at all, get on the phone. It's OK to ask for help.
4. Avoid dosing yourself with "polypharmacy" (many different over-the-counter preparations). Some of them singly, but especially in combination, are dangerous if overused or used for the wrong indications. Also, follow the dosage instructions on the bottles. They invariably are conservative in nature, which will help prevent problems.
5. Use the emergency room for true emergencies, not for ordinary care. These are, nowadays, overcrowded, expensive, and occasionally hazardous to your health. Of course, if you have a real emergency and you can't get right through to your doctor, you'd better go to the emergency room.
6. The following section will be useful to you in your own medical care. I have listed, with commentary, the items that are prudent to have on hand. Don't forget, though, to keep these medicines away from children who may be harmed by their unsupervised use.

Medical Supplies for Your Medicine Chest

These are some of the simple medications and supplies that are handy to have around. Generics, if available, are usually OK.

1. *Analgesics* such as aspirin, acetaminophen (Tylenol), ibuprofen (Advil and many other brands). These are useful in case of pain of

any sort. They are also useful for fever. Note that aspirin and ibuprofen are NSAIDS (nonsteroidal anti-inflammatory drugs) and are potentially harmful to the upper gastrointestinal tract and kidneys (especially in older people). The major cause of gastrointestinal bleeding is these medications, not ulcers. Acetaminophen is safest for the stomach but too much can harm the liver (particularly when taken with alcohol). A new class of NSAIDs called the COX-2 inhibitors has been developed (e.g., Celebrex®). These drugs are thought to be safer than the other NSAIDs because they seem to spare the gastrointestinal tract. They are far more expensive, however, and their long-term safety and efficacy are unknown.

2. *Antihistamines* such as Chlortrimeton® or Benadryl® (and many others). These are useful for any kind of allergic reactions (skin, nasal, or other). They do not help colds, however. They can cause drowsiness. The new nondrowsy kind (Hismanal®, Claritin®, and so on) require a prescription.

3. *Bicarbonate of soda* (baking soda or "bicarb"). *Great stuff!* It is inexpensive and marvelous for soothing skin or eye irritations or burns, for wet compresses, as a gargle, mouthwash, even an antacid (it is not advisable to use it for this, other than occasionally, because the sodium content is very high).

4. *Cough medicine.* The only nonprescription cough suppressant of note is dextromethorphan (Robitussin-DM® and others). It usually comes in combination with other, probably ineffective but harmless, ingredients such as antihistamines and expectorants (guaifenesin). It's worth trying every four hours or so, but hot liquids (soup, tea) may be just as good. Potent cough suppressants contain either codeine or its derivatives, which need a prescription.

5. *Decongestants* are helpful for a stuffy nose. The most common are pseudoephedrine (Sudafed® and generics) and phenylephrine. These, if used in large doses, may be overstimulating and may cause nervousness and insomnia. Topical decongestants (sprays or drops) such as oxymetazoline (Afrin® and generics) will open a clogged nose for a while, but if used too often or for too long may cause rebound con-

gestion and nasal addiction. The liquid applied to a cotton ball and inserted into the nose may also stop stubborn nosebleeds. Saline sprays or drops (Ayr® or Ocean® nasal spray) are useful and less apt to cause trouble than the decongestants.

6. *Antinausea* medicines are useful for various gastrointestinal upsets including motion sickness. The most commonly used are Dramamine® or Bonine® (or generics).

7. *Antacids* are useful for heartburn, indigestion, and various gastrointestinal discomforts. They are usually aluminum magnesium (Maalox®, Mylanta®) or calcium types (Tums®, Rolaids®). Gaviscon® may be useful for nocturnal heartburn, especially since it tends to float on the stomach contents and bathes the lower end of the esophagus, which needs protection from acid. Generally, these drugs are harmless and worth a try. Sometimes they are combined with simethicone, which is supposed to break up gas bubbles.

8. *Acid blockers.* These have just been released (1995) from prescription requirements (Tagamet®, Pepcid®, Zantac®). They are potent and quite expensive, but they are true suppressors of acid production. They have some potential side effects and they should not be used for very long without your doctor's knowledge and approval.

9. *Laxatives and stool softeners.* A large variety exist and are OK if used only on occasion and *in the absence of abdominal pain.* The safest types are the bulk laxatives (Metamucil®, Konsyl®, Citracel®) which, when taken with lots of water, are safe and stimulate the colon by simple distention. This form of soluble fiber (psyllium seed or methylcellulose) also may help in lowering cholesterol, an extra advantage. Other laxatives work by stimulating or irritating the colonic wall to a greater or lesser extent. Mild ones such as senna extracts (Senokot®, Feen-a-Mint®), salts (milk of magnesia), and docusate (Doxidan®) are safe, if used only on occasion. Stool softeners (Colace® and generics) are basically detergents and have no appreciable risk.

10. *Diarrhea medicines* are of two basic types, adsorbents such as kaolin (Kaopectate®) and bismuth preparations (Pepto-Bismol), and

smooth muscle bowel relaxers such as Lomotil® and Imodium. Stronger ones such as opium compounds (paragoric) are prescription-controlled medicines. The safest and most effective ones are the bismuth preparations (good old Pepto-Bismol) in proper doses (every hour or so until the diarrhea stops). One warning—bismuth compounds may turn the tongue and the feces black due to the combination with sulfur in the gastrointestinal tract. (Scary to see but harmless.) Imodium and Lomotil stop cramps and diarrhea by temporarily paralyzing the bowel muscle. This may not be a good thing if, for instance, toxins or viruses need to be eliminated or adsorbed. It is best to try the adsorbents first.

11. *Topical agents* (applied to the skin):
    Antiseptics. Germ-killing substances are highly touted but are mostly ineffective, or at least hardly better than plain soap and water cleansing. Antibacterial soaps, such as Phisohex® and others, may be useful for chronic or recurrent skin infections such as boils or acne, because they leave a residue of an antiseptic medicine (hexachlorophene) on the skin. Iodine compounds, Zephiran® compounds, hydrogen peroxide, alcohol, and so on may be more psychotherapy than bactericidal, but unless there is skin sensitivity, they can't hurt.
    Antibiotic creams or ointments such as Neosporin® or Polysporin® are useful for infection-prone open wounds such as abrasions or shaving cuts or burns.
    Fungicidal creams or ointments are effective for athlete's foot, ringworm, or other fungus infections (if you know what they are, fine; if you don't, check with your doctor). These include such preparations as Lotrimin®, Aftate®, Desenex®, and Tinactin®, among others.
    Dandruff shampoos such as Selsun® or salicylate (Head & Shoulders®) and others including tar or sulfur preparations may relieve scalp seborrhea.
    Aluminum acetate (Domeboro®) powder can be diluted into an excellent solution for compresses and soaks for infected or wet inflamed areas. It is germicidal, soothing, and drying. This is worth knowing about.

Rubbing alcohol (70% isopropyl) is a good, all-around cleanser and antiseptic. It removes oily dirt better than water. But don't drink it! It also, when diluted half and half with water, makes a nice cooling rub for the fevered body.

Liniments. Aching joints and muscles may be relieved somewhat by these counterirritating substances, liquid or cream. These are usually methylsalicylate (oil of wintergreen) or menthol based (Mineral Ice®).

Emollients and moisturizers. These are very useful for itchy, dry skin, a particular problem in hot, dry, sunbaked times of the year in various parts of the world. Most are okay—my favorites are Acid-Mantle®, Alpha Keri®, Lubriderm®, and Skin-So-Soft®. By the way, I don't know whether this latter preparation works as an insect repellent as some people, including my wife, claim.

Cortisone-type creams. Forty years ago, an old dermatologist told me his deathbed secret of dermatology: "If it's wet, dry it. If it's dry, wet it. In any case, put cortisone on it." Cortisone is actually a hormone produced by the adrenal gland. Its discovery, as a "wonder drug" back in the 1940s, heralded a new age of endocrinology (science of glands of internal secretion) and therapy. The stuff was an incredible anti-inflammatory medicine that had multiple applications. It is a major treatment for all types of skin inflammations and allergies. Over the years, more and more potent cortisone-like medicines have developed, but the only ones available without a prescription contain hydrocortisone, ½ percent or 1 percent. Stronger preparations need professional guidance in their use. They may cause skin thinning and other problems. The 1 percent hydrocortisone creams are great for insect bites, poison ivy or oak, and many other inflammations. They should not be used on actual infections, however. They may aggravate these.

Sunscreens. Very important (see section on skin problems). They provide protection from ultraviolet rays, which can cause severe burning and even more severe, long-term complications. These substances are either based on PABA (para-amino benzoic acid), to

Figure 4-1: THINGS YOU SHOULD KEEP IN YOUR MEDICINE CHEST

Acid Blockers (Tagamet, Pepcid, Zantac)

Adhesive tape

Afrin nasal spray (generic available)

Analgesics (aspirin, acetaminophen, ibuprofen): for pain and/or fever

Antacids (Mylanta, Maalox, Gaviscon)

Antibiotic cream or ointment

Antidiarrheals (Pepto-Bismol, Imodium)

Antihistamines: for allergies of all kinds

Antinausea (seasick) remedies (Dramamine, Bonine)

Antiseptic soap (Phisohex)

Athlete's foot fungus cream

Band-Aid® adhesive bandages

Bicarbonate of soda

Cough medicine: for cough suppression or expectorant (guaifenesin)

Dandruff shampoo

Decongestants: for nasal congestion, colds, and allergies

Domeboro

Elastic (e.g., Ace®) bandages (2" and/or 4")

Eyedrops: artificial tears

1% Hydrocortisone cream

Laxative: bulk, milk of magnesia, senna

Liniment

Moisturizing cream

Rubbing alcohol

Saline nasal spray

Sterile gauze pads

Sunscreen

Thermometer

which some people are sensitive, or use other active ingredients, but range in strength from minimum to maximum, with SPF (sun protection factor) numbering from 4 to 45. Use them!

Eyedrops. The redness-relieving drops consist mainly of blood vessel constrictors which "bleach" the whites of the eyes and are only of cosmetic help. The only eyedrops and salves that can be unhesitatingly recommended are those which help prevent dryness. This is a problem that is ubiquitous and increases as one ages, particularly in dry climates. These substances, known usually as artificial tears or lubricants, do work to keep the eye membranes moist. Eyewashes are generally ineffective—instead, use good old baking soda in cool, moist compresses (about 1 teaspoon to 1 pint of warm water). If a red eye does not improve within a day of this treatment, call the doctor.

12. *Other supplies:*

A good *thermometer.* Fancy digital ones are available and accurate but old-fashioned, inexpensive mercury ones are fine. Don't forget to shake it down before using. Take your temperature before calling the doctor for flu or other suspected infections. It saves time.

Band-Aids sterile gauze pads (2" x 2" to 4") are very handy to keep around.

Don't forget: follow the dose instructions on the packages. First do (yourself) no harm.

DR. DASHE'S TIPS FOR HEALTH MAINTENANCE

1. Most ailments are transient or trivial and will go away naturally.

2. Make yourself familiar with the signs and symptoms of illnesses that can be easily handled at home without a doctor's intervention.

3. The intensity of the ailment is the most important criterion for calling the doctor. If the pain is unbearable, get medical help immediately.

4. Duration of symptoms is the next important indicator. If the sickness lasts longer than three days, a call to the doctor is in order.

5. Is it getting better, or worse? If you're not getting any better after a while call the doctor. The three day rule applies here, too.

6. Severe pain, especially in the chest region warrants a call for help.

7. Milder discomfort, including occasional headaches, heartburn, cramps associated with gas or diarrhea, or musculoskeletal aches, usually respond to analgesics and time.

8. Bleeding from any orifice is usually alarming and, unless the cause is obvious, will need medical attention.

9. Keep a well-stocked and rational medicine chest for ordinary use. There are many simple over-the-counter remedies which are very helpful and, incidentally, weren't even available to the grand physicians of yesteryear.

10. Knowledge of your body and a working knowledge of minor complaints and symptoms will help you save the doctor some time in some instances or save your life in others.

PART II

Review of Systems:
How Things Work

The following chapters will deal with the various functioning parts that make up the whole of our physical being. A great deal of information must be covered; clearly even more must be left out because of the various constraints inherent in a book of this type. I have chosen to emphasize the matters that seem to have been most germane to my male patients over the years. For instance, although molecular biology and genetic research and engineering are the cutting edges of medicine these days, backache, hair loss, and safe sex are what concern most of us, so I'll sacrifice the space-age scientific lecturing in favor of the practical side. I will conclude the book with chapters on aging and the unique status that manhood confers upon us.

Chapter 5

BONES AND MUSCLES

"Why on earth," I wondered to myself, "did I begin this section with bones and muscles?" One has to start somewhere, but this was almost an automatic choice. Then I remembered that's how I started medical school. To this day, medical school begins with the skeleton and the muscle anatomy. The ancient physicians, too, considered this primary and the anatomic drawings of Leonardo da Vinci, Vesalius, and others are classics attesting to the fascination with the stature and movement of the human body. To us as men, the ability to be upright and to move with ease and agility is an incredibly important matter. Being laid low with a backache or a bad knee is not only painful, it is demoralizing to the ego, even at times disastrous, if your livelihood depends upon your mobility. We need to know something about our structure and its functions and potential dysfunctions.

The bony skeleton, as you know, is the sturdy framework which supports our physical structure. The bones, some 270-plus in all, are constructed of tough materials, namely calcium salts embedded in a protein matrix. Built around the axial skeleton, which is the spine, are the skull, ribs, shoulders, and hip girdles to which the upper and lower extremities are joined with movable joints called articulations (Figure 5-1).

Figure 5-1: THE HUMAN SKELETON

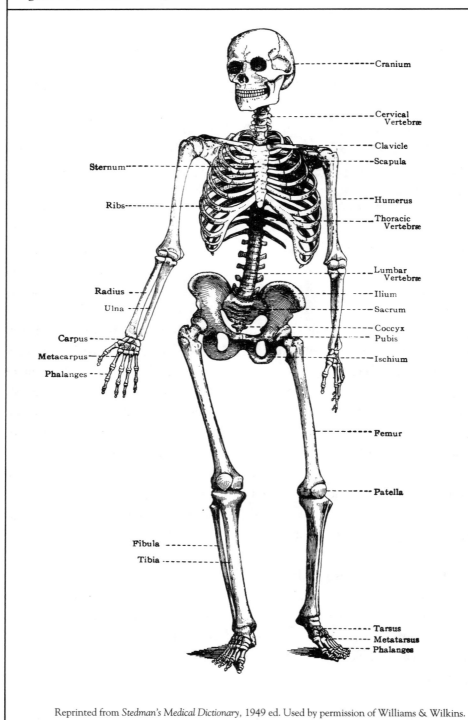

Cranium

Cervical Vertebræ

Clavicle

Scapula

Sternum

Humerus

Ribs

Thoracic Vertebræ

Lumbar Vertebræ

Radius

Ilium

Ulna

Sacrum

Coccyx

Carpus

Pubis

Metacarpus

Ischium

Phalanges

Femur

Patella

Fibula

Tibia

Tarsus

Metatarsus

Phalanges

Reprinted from *Stedman's Medical Dictionary*, 1949 ed. Used by permission of Williams & Wilkins.

The separate bones articulate with one another as a movable joint by means of tendons and ligaments, which are tough, white sheets of connective tissue. The joints may be freely movable. There are hinge joints such as fingers, pivot joints such as the elbow, and ball-and-socket joints like shoulders and hips which have multidirectional capabilities. Some joints are only slightly movable, such as the spine (vertebrae). Where bones touch each other they have elegant, smooth surfaces which act as permanent lubricated plates called cartilages (tough, rubbery, smooth, white structures which protect the hard bones from grating on one another). The joints are motivated by the action, contraction, and/or relaxation of the muscles, which are attached to the bones by the tough, white sinews called tendons. Bursas are the lubricated sheaths that enclose the tendons and ligaments and permit smooth "sliding" of these structures during muscle movement. Movements are produced, depending upon the nature of the joint and the points of attachment of the muscles. For instance, you flex the forearm (bend it toward you) by the contraction of the biceps muscle and the simultaneous relaxation of the opposite group (triceps). Extension of the forearm (bending it away from you) occurs with just the reverse of these motions (Figure 5-2). The muscles, some 500-plus of them, are marvelous mechanisms themselves. They may be flexors or extensors or both, depending upon the structure they serve. And even more incredibly, they move at the almost instantaneous command of the brain and spinal cord (central nervous system) via the motor nerves that supply them. The muscles consist of bundles of fibers which have the ability to shorten or lengthen with proper nerve stimulation.

With this understanding of anatomy, we can discuss and define the ailments that may bother our musculoskeletal system. Some definitions:

1. Fracture—when a bone breaks. Simple fractures imply a simple bone break with or without displacement of the ends. The much more serious compound fracture means that a bone fragment has broken through the skin and infection may result. Comminuted fractures are also more serious, since the bone has broken into more than one fragment.

Figure 5-2: MUSCLES OF THE ARM

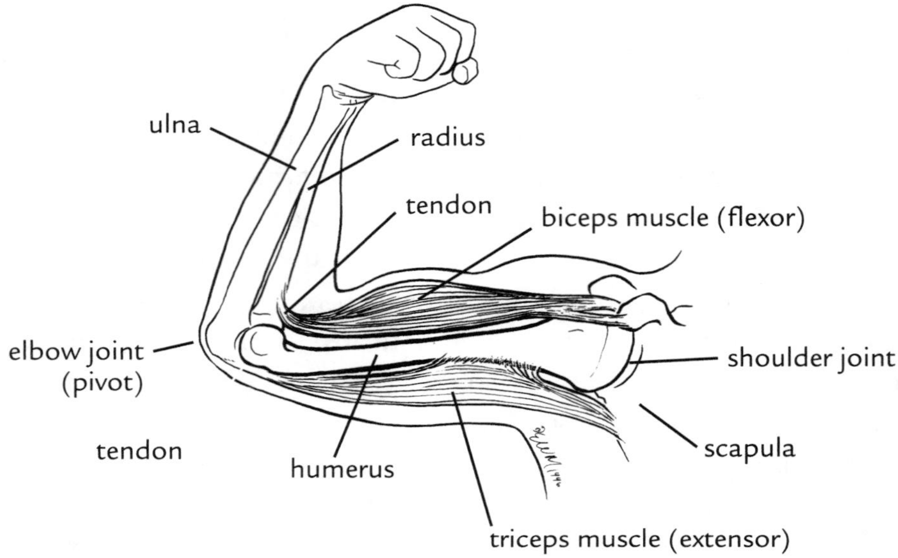

Illustration by Elizabeth Weadon Massari.

2. Dislocation—the joint and ligaments are disrupted and torn, without fracture, but the two ends of the joints are separated and must be put back into place to function.
3. Sprain—this means a tear of a ligament, tendon, or muscle of varying degree, but usually not a total separation.
4. Strain—this is a lesser sprain, probably a few fibers of muscle or ligament are torn, but without separation.
5. -itis—means inflammation, for example, arthritis = an inflamed joint, tendonitis = an inflamed tendon, myositis = an inflamed muscle or muscles, fibrositis = a general term meaning, usually, inflammation of a ligament, tendon, or other connective tissue.
6. -algia—means pain, with or without other damage, for example, myalgia = painful muscle, arthralgia = painful joint.
7. -osis—means a chronic or continual condition or problem. You can tack any prefix to it, if it's an ongoing condition.

Now we can review the more common important diseases that affect the human musculoskeletal system.

Common Problems—
From Bottom to Top

Feet

Considering the burdens placed on them, the feet do a great job. Bear in mind that our nearest primate relatives, the great apes, use all four extremities in standing and walking. Bipedal mammals are unusual in nature. The upright stance has given us not only advantageous height, but also the free use of our hands, putting us pretty much on top of the evolutionary ladder, along with the boxing kangaroos.

Feet do take a beating, not only from our weight bearing but also from the enormous increased stresses associated with walking, running, and jogging in shoes that are designed more for fashion than for anatomy and function. It is little consolation that women are far worse than men in this regard. In women's shoes, heel elevation forces the forefoot down into the pointy, funnel-like toe of the shoe, deforming the foot over the years and guaranteeing bunion formation, hammer toes, and corns. Men's dress shoes have been generally better designed and the aforementioned deformities are less common and are usually associated with congenital defects, usual wear and tear, and changes caused by arthritis. Proper shoes, those that have enough room for the toes and good support in the instep, cost more but are worth the expense, particularly shoes used for running or other sports.

Bunions are inflamed protuberances at the junction of the big toe and the foot. Corns are calluses of the upper side of the small joints of the toes, caused by pressure and rubbing against a shoe. Plantar warts are true warts that form on the pressure-bearing points of the sole of the foot. They are very painful and hard to get rid of.

Once difficulties have developed, treatment may be required by a podiatrist or orthopedist who specializes in foot problems. You should ask for a referral from your personal doctor. Some podiatrists are too quick to perform immediate major surgery. Before doing anything, however, invest in well-fitting, comfortable shoes.

Ankles

This joint between the foot and leg has movement limited to two planes; upward and downward is the major one, and side-to-side a more limited motion. Tough ligaments hold this joint in place. Too much of a sidewise twist may tear these ligaments to a greater or lesser degree, producing the common affliction known as ankle sprain. The degree of tear, from a few broken ligament fibers to a complete tear, determines the time and amount of disability. Almost always these tears will heal if the joint is splinted and weight bearing avoided for enough time, up to six to eight weeks in severe cases. Only rarely is surgery (to sew up the ligaments) needed. A severe sprain will cause swelling, pain, and black and blue marks from bleeding under the skin. Immediate treatment should consist of elevation of the foot, icing, wrapping the ankle with an elastic bandage and, if pain and swelling are severe, calling the doctor. X-rays may be necessary to exclude fracture. The end of the fibula, the skinny, outer bone of the leg (the inner, thicker one is the tibia) forms one side of the mortise joint that is the ankle and is subject to fracture in association with severe sprain-type injury. Orthopedic treatment is required and consists, usually, of casting. In any case, avoidance of weight bearing for a variable period is necessary. Crutches are handy supporting devices that, at the same time, allow you to appreciate more fully the wonderful work of the normal lower extremities.

Legs

The two leg bones (tibia and fibula) are surrounded by strong muscles confined by tough membranes to three compartments. The rear, or calf, compartment contains the strong calf muscles (gastrocnemius and soleus) that attach to the ankle bone with the famous Achilles' tendon. These powerful muscles permit us to toe dance and jump. They also will tear (or their tendons will) if we get too playful. This is a sad, incapacitating situation, requiring crutches and a cast and occasionally reparative surgery.

Less onerous and more common are leg cramps, caused by muscle spasms. They are rarely due to metabolic (mineral depletion) cause. They may be caused by over- or underuse of the legs, but they are usually easily handled by gentle stretching of leg muscles. For instance, keeping the feet flat on the floor, body straight, arm's length from the wall, slowly bring the chest to the wall, feel the stretch in the legs, wait a few seconds for relaxation to occur, and remain in this position for a count of five. Don't bounce—do it slowly. This is especially good at bedtime to prevent nocturnal cramps. It works better than drugs of any kind.

The front compartments on each side of the tibia (shinbone) contain muscle bundles and tendons that can become inflamed and ache and cramp. These painful symptoms are called shin splints and are usually brought on by vigorous leg activity. Treatment is rest, massage, minor analgesics, and hot or cold applications.

Knees

The knee is a limited-motion joint located between the tibia and the bottom of the thighbone (femur). It is held in its position by strong ligaments (the cruciate ligaments), both external and internal, which assure the flexion and extension of the leg. Twisting motion is severely limited but if forced, injury, especially tearing of the cruciate ligaments, often happens. Even more often, the lubricating cartilage plates (the menisci), where the two bones meet and articulate, are torn by adverse motion. The knee, so important to our gait, is terribly delicate. Even if uninjured, knees wear out with time, become arthritic, and often cause incapacitation because of the pain and swelling produced by walking and weight bearing. Fortunately, orthopedic surgery has done well in dealing with knee problems. Arthroscopic surgery is used regularly for both diagnosis and treatment of knee problems. This is surgery performed through a small, lighted tube inserted under the skin. No major cutting is required and it is much less incapacitating to the patient. Results are usually favorable. Trouble-causing substances such as bits of broken cartilage and arthritic bone and other debris can be removed, surfaces smoothed and planed, and recently, even new cartilage cells grafted in place. Ligaments may be repaired, although for the worst tears a more extensive "open" operation with grafting of donor ligaments may be performed. Sports star Ed O'Bannon of UCLA and the NBA had such a career-saving procedure recently. In prior years his career would have been ended. Perhaps even more amazing is knee replacement surgery. Techniques and prostheses have become so good lately that the results give credence to the "Bionic Man" stories.

Hips

The femur, the largest long bone of the body, extends from the knee to the hip, where it connects with the pelvic bone (ileum) socket and joins the rest of the body. The femur is a massively strong bone surrounded by thick, powerful muscles (the thigh muscles, called the vasti because of their bulk). Its weakest point is at the neck where the ball and socket joint of the hip articulates. The ball is the hip, the socket is the pelvis. The narrow neck from the ball to the body of the femur is thus subject to major geometric stresses and is the common site of hip fractures. Hip fractures often used to be death sentences to people. They took forever to heal by themselves and required total bed care for months or years (an intolerable and frequently lethal state, particularly for the aged). Again, bionics have changed all that. Hip replacement surgery is effective, rapid, and amazing, used not only for fractures but for the just-as-common incapacitating hip arthritis (once called malum coxae senilis or "sick hips of the old"). The misery and danger of hip disease has, to a large part, been mitigated by modern surgery, another incredible advance.

Spine

The spine is the bane of the vertical animal. Veterinarians tell me that backaches and ruptured discs do not occur in our four-footed brethren unless they happen to be beasts of burden (horses) or bred to have abnormally long back length (dachshunds and basset hounds). Consider this in terms of simple physics. When upright, the spine must bear not only the weight of the body (and what might be added by carrying something) but also the tension of the guy-wire-like muscles of the spine, which contract to keep the spine from collapsing. The actual pressure borne by the spine is multiplied when one bends over, such as to pick up a parcel. Therefore, it is important to squat rather than bend when picking up something. Between each vertebra (seven cervical, twelve thoracic, five lumbar) there is a cushion called a disc. These are soft, pulpy, almost liquid cores surrounded and kept in place by a tough ligament. When this ligament, which is under considerable pressure, weakens and bulges or breaks (ruptured disc), pressure from extruded disc material may press on the nerves emanating from the spine and innervating the muscles and sensory nerves of the extremities. These unpleasant events occur most commonly in the lumbar (lower back) and cervical (neck) disc spaces since these are the most mobile of the vertebrae and are subject to the greatest stress. The actual symptoms are most commonly due to pressure on the peripheral nerves and not the spinal cord itself (except, rarely, in the neck—see later section on the neck). Low back pain itself, therefore, is almost never due to ruptured disc. Disc pain is usually manifested by pain radiating down the legs, sciatica, which is pressure on the sciatic nerve, the longest nerve in the body, extending from the posterior (back part) of the hip down through the buttock and back of the leg to the foot.

Back pain itself, without sciatica, is usually due to muscle sprain or strain and may usually be handled by rest, heat, gentle massage, gentle stretching exercises while lying down, and oral analgesics. It has recently been determined, by careful controlled studies, that medical or chiropractic measures offer little help in the management of backache. Indeed, a recent investigation revealed that getting up and resuming gentle nonstressful normal activity may actually hasten recovery. Prolonged bed rest is no longer recommended. Another recent medical bombshell is the incidental finding of many instances of bulging discs when MRI studies of the spine in asymptomatic people were reviewed. This raises the question of the significance of the "disc syndrome." Probably, especially in cases of severe rupture where disc material is really dislocated and is seen pressing on a nerve, there is a cause and effect. Even in most of these situations, time and conservative management is the answer. Surgical removal of the offending disc is rarely necessary, but in the worst instances where not only pain but muscle weakness occurs, surgical intervention may be dramatically helpful. This surgery should not be taken lightly or without good consultation, for complications and failure, though uncommon in the best surgical hands, may be catastrophic and lead to prolonged disability.

A word about exercise. I have already mentioned that certain exercises, for instance weight bearing and "pounding" exercises such as jogging, may aggravate the back. Some exercises, by virtue of their back and abdominal muscle-building nature, may help prevent stiffening and pain in the back (the "abs" are the front guy-wires of the skeleton). These exercises are generally done while lying down and may consist of simple head and leg raises and "crunches." I strongly urge people who suffer from backaches and stiffness, particularly in the morning, to do the following stretch before getting out of bed. First, pull each knee up to the chin, keeping it there for ten or fifteen seconds; then both knees together to the chin for ten or fifteen seconds. Repeat two or three times.

Neck

It's amazing how heavy the head is—about 20 pounds or more in the normal adult even without worries. The neck is quite mobile, too, and simple maintenance of the upright posture creates stresses on the neck joints, discs, and muscles—similar to the back. Also, as in the back, x-ray studies of the neck in people over the age of forty-five invariably show disc and arthritic changes in the cervical vertebrae. The manifestations of this cervical neck disease are almost always related to pressure on the nerves to the upper extremities, with pain, numbness, and tingling being most common. Weakness of the upper extremities, fortunately, is rare. But when it occurs it requires neurosurgical consultation because it is a serious and potentially disabling disorder. Actual cervical spinal cord damage is almost never seen in the absence of trauma or rough manipulation of the head or neck. This, of course, is a major medical emergency and requires immediate expert management. For the usual and very common neckache, with or without the radiating nerve symptoms, conservative treatment is helpful. Again, heat, massage, gentle strengthening and stretching exercises, and analgesics are in order. Also, in severe cases, particularly when the onset is acute (generally signaling an injury or sprain has occurred) a well-fitting, soft, supporting neck collar may be helpful, at least to keep the head upright and prevent bending and twisting. A cervical pillow—that is, a pillow that keeps the head supported but the neck straight, may be very helpful for sleep at night. Neck traction is of questionable value, and a chiropractor's manipulation is a definite no-no.

Shoulders

Moving to the upper extremities we come to one of the most mobile joints in the body, the shoulder. It is an elegant ball and socket that assures our athletic skills as well as permits us to hunt, throw, gather, drink, and hug. This was brought home to me in no uncertain terms one day after I had given a glorious demonstration of the one-handed basketball push shot. The next day I was unable to raise my arm from my body because of the excruciating pain this simple movement produced. I turned myself in to the neighborhood orthopedist and after some preliminary x-rays was informed that I was the owner of a case of shoulder bursitis. Bursitis, if you recall, is an inflamed tendon sheath. In this case, it was my supraspinatus muscle tendon, part of the rotator cuff, which is activated when raising one's arm straight out and doing one-handed push shots. Shoulder bursitis, as any type, can be brought on by repetitive stress to a tendon. This happens a lot with this joint, as well as the elbow (see below). Treatment consists of rest and immobilization (arm sling), anti-inflammatory drugs (aspirin and NSAIDs), heat or cold (both may work), and sometimes a cortisone injection into the tendon sheath. I was well again within the week. My kids, in the meanwhile, had taken up soccer.

Rotator cuff tears are a more serious problem. "Rotator cuff" refers to the muscular and fibrous layers over the shoulder joint that form a continuous cuff, keeping the ball and socket of the humerus (upper arm bone) and scapula in place and permitting the rotating motion of the shoulder. This is a key structure and a tear or other disruption of this cuff usually results in painful disability regarding shoulder motion, particularly elevation of the arm greater than 90 degrees. Treatment consists of rest with a sling, anti-inflammatory drugs, and special exercises (best handled, at least at first, by a physical therapist). If conservative measures are ineffective, surgical repair, either open or arthroscopic, may be required.

Other common shoulder problems are separation and fracture of the collar bone (clavicle). Separation means tearing of the ligament that binds the clavicle to the shoulder. These bones are tied together by tough ligaments and may be torn when one falls squarely upon one's shoulder as can occur in sports, and in my own case karate practice. With a more severe fall, the clavicle itself may fracture. Both situations are painful, but both usually respond nicely to simple binding of the shoulders with a "figure eight" splint.

Dislocation of the shoulder joint occurs when the head of the humerus, which is a ball-like structure, is forcefully pulled or knocked out of its socket. The capsule of the joint, which actually is incorporated with the rotator cuff, is torn as well most of the time. The pain is usually excruciating until the ball is replaced, which is usually easy to do after administering strong pain medicine. This is a very dramatic event to watch, with the orthopedist removing his shoe, placing his foot in the poor victim's armpit, and yanking the arm until the ball plops back into its socket. Pain relief is usually quite dramatic as well. Healing may take place without surgery, but frequently the shoulder capsule must be stitched to prevent recurrent dislocations.

In almost all cases, orthopedic examination and treatment is warranted with shoulder problems, certainly if pain and/or disablement persists after two or three days of conservative home measures (rest, sling, heat, cold, oral analgesics).

Elbow

Between the upper arm and forearm, the elbow joint provides multipurpose movements: flexion, extension, and rotation. It's also useful for a leaning point. Too much elbow leaning may lead to a swollen, inflamed bursa at the point of the elbow (also known as bartenders', psychiatrists', or judges', disease). This ulnar bursitis is painful and unsightly, but usually responds well to removal of fluid and injection of cortisone followed by wrapping with an elastic bandage.

The other type of elbow bursitis is referred to as "tennis elbow" and is caused by any repetitive motion of an elbow tendon in its sheath. Treatment is similar to the other types of bursitis mentioned: rest, anti-inflammatory drugs, analgesics, and/or cortisone injection.

Wrist and Hand

We conclude the voyage up the skeleton to the ultimate tools, the wrist and hand. The utility of this has given our species, under the direction of the human brain, dominion over other life forms. All is within our grasp, as it were, considering the opposable thumb. Anatomy and function of the hand is special enough even to rate its own superspecialty in orthopedics. Practitioners of this art are, in my experience, some of the most skillful surgeons in practice, and well they must be because the mechanisms are delicate and precise. Much is written about the hand and wrist but I shall limit my discussion to a few of the most common conditions, all of which require professional expertise in management.

Fractures of the delicate bones of the hand and wrist are common, especially those caused by falling on the outstretched hand. Particularly in younger men, the occurrence of a hidden or occult fracture of the scaphoid bone of the wrist may not appear on a regular x-ray until weeks after the event. So if pain persists after such a fall, even with no apparent deformity on the x-ray, this fracture must be considered and follow-up studies done, including bone scans, which are far more sensitive. If untreated, carpal (wrist) scaphoid fractures lead to a permanently painful, arthritic wrist. In older people, the same type of fall usually leads to an easily diagnosed and immediately treated "Colles" type fracture, which is diagnosed by a typical bent-up deformity of the wrist and lower forearm.

Another common problem is carpal tunnel syndrome. The median nerve of the hand, which innervates the muscles and sensation of most of the hand, travels through a bony tunnel on the palm side of the wrist. The tunnel is enclosed by a tough ligament or fascia. Narrowing of this tunnel from any cause, such as recurrent injury, arthritic change of the bones of the wrist, or soft-tissue swelling, will cause compression of the nerve and symptoms of tingling and numbness of the hand as well as loss of power in the hand muscles and fingers.

Diagnosis is made by examination and electric nerve testing. Treatment is usually successful; with surgical release of the tight band or sometimes anti-inflammatory medicines or injection of cortisone.

Dupuytren's contracture is another common problem, often seen after the age of forty, and may be associated with diabetes and, oddly, excessive alcohol use. Usually, however, the cause is unknown. The condition is manifested by scarring and contraction of the palm of the hand to a greater or lesser degree. In most cases, it is mild and not incapacitating. It just appears to be a tough flat scar on the palm. At worst, the shortening of the scar tissue pulls the fingers in toward the palm, interfering with hand function. The treatment, if needed, is surgical removal of the scar tissue.

Now that we've made the trip from the tip of the toe to the tip of the hand, I will conclude this chapter with some remarks about generalized musculoskeletal disorders.

Osteoporosis

Osteoporosis describes loss of bone density, usually of metabolic cause, and is due to loss of bone matrix and the calcium salts embedded therein. Fortunately, it is a relatively rare occurrence in men. It is very common in women, particularly postmenopausal or hormone-deficient ones. The reason for this difference is simple. Men do not generally suffer from severe loss of the anabolic (tissue-building) male hormone, testosterone, until very late in life. Women do lose their anabolic hormone, estrogen, relatively early, after menopause. (This is one reason that more women are now urged to go on estrogen replacement after menopause or other cause of loss of hormone.) Osteoporosis in a male, therefore, needs medical evaluation and treatment. Various tumors (parathyroid, some cancers) or metabolic disease (hyperthyroidism) may cause this, but probably the most common cause in males is use of cortisone-type medicine (steroids) for other diseases. These drugs are catabolic (tissue-wasting) hormones and may cause serious bone loss with attendant danger of easy fracture. Of course, advanced age (over age seventy-five) is another potential cause. Ordinarily, calcium supplementation in the healthy, active male is not necessary, but some authorities advise about 1 to 2 gms per day in men over age sixty-five. There are other potent osteoporosis remedies available, if necessary, but medical evaluation is needed before such use. These include the bone-building hormones (testosterone, calcitonin) and a newer class of drugs known as the biphosphonates, Fosamax® and Didronel®.

Arthritis

I have previously mentioned that the suffix *itis* is usually applied to conditions of inflammation, acute rather than chronic. In the case of arthritis, therefore, the joints are inflamed, sometimes acutely, but even more often on an intermittent or ongoing basis. Inflammation is a term denoting a condition of painful, swollen, hot, and reddened tissues. Inflammation actually is a defense mechanism of the body. Without this we would not survive. When the body tissues are attacked by invaders from outside (bacteria or viruses) or within (antibodies), the response is an all-out counteroffensive using cellular (white blood cells) and chemical defenders. We perceive this response as inflammation. The battle may rage in any part of the body. For example, in the skin a boil or abscess may form (remember heat, pain, redness, swelling). In a joint, we have arthritis.

There are many types and causes of arthritis and it is not possible here to describe them all. Arthritis needs to be diagnosed and treated properly by your doctor.

Most common, and to some extent probably affecting all of us, is osteoarthritis. This is also called degenerative joint disease. It is manifested by chronic breakdown of cartilage in the joints leading to pain, stiffness, and swelling. It is the garden variety wear and tear that occurs with the ongoing use of our bones and joints. Things wear out, and our bodies are no different, though happily, they are tougher than most man-made machines. Of course the rougher and longer the use, the sooner and worse the wear. There is a genetic propensity to this (as with most everything else); there seems to be a vague inherited tendency regarding the severity and time of onset of osteoarthritis. Certainly, however, major use and abuse of the skeletal system will bring it on prematurely. This is why professional athletes tend toward early cripplehood and retirement in their twenties to forties. Interestingly, although osteoarthritis creates deformities (of the "knobby" variety) and pain, there may be no correlation between the two. Occasionally one sees major deformity (especially in hands) with little or no pain, and vice versa. The difference is in the amount of inflammation, the severity of which varies with the individual. Osteoarthritis is a variable, sometimes painful, sometimes disabling, but nonfatal disease.

There are a number of far more serious forms of arthritis. These are systemic (or total body) disorders with joint manifestations a major feature. There are too many to enumerate here but they include such diseases as rheumatoid arthritis, lupus, gout, and scleroderma. All of these require professional medical attention and have specific diagnostic and therapeutic components.

One arthritic disorder that bears particular interest for readers of this book, however, is gout. An ancient and fascinating disease historically, it is an ailment mainly of the male and is rarely seen in women. It tends to be hereditary. So many prominent men suffered from gout that it came to be associated over the centuries with being rich and famous. But fame is not a prerequisite. It can happen to anyone who has a high level of uric acid in the blood. Uric acid is a product of the metabolic digestion of our cellular nuclei. We are constantly turning over many of our tissues, destroying the old, worn-out cells and replacing them with new ones. Uric acid is a waste product of this process that is transported by the blood to the kidneys, which then excretes this substance into the urine (hence the term "uric"). The stuff is soluble in blood up to a certain level. If this is exceeded, the material tends to crystallize, like rock candy in a sugary solution. Unfortunately, uric acid crystals are tiny needle-like particles which have the propensity to cause a violent inflammatory reaction when deposited in joints. This is the cause of gouty arthritis, which causes joints to be violently painful, red, hot, and swollen. Any joint may be affected, but most commonly it is the big toe or foot. The reason for this is simply that uric acid crystallizes first in tissues that are slightly acidic. Any type of minor injury, such as stubbing one's toe, will cause a slightly acid tissue change which may precipitate an acute gouty attack. Uric acid can crystallize in other tissues as well, causing "tophi" or whitish bumps under the skin, particularly hands and ears. When uric acid crystallizes in the kidneys or ureters, stones may form which can cause excruciating pain. The only good thing about gout is that it is easily diagnosed by measurement of the uric acid blood levels and it is also generally easily treated with medicines such as anti-inflammatory drugs (NSAIDs or colchicine). Drugs such as allopurinol, which prevents uric acid formation, or probenecid (Benemid®), which hastens excretion, are used to lower blood uric acid levels. Certain foods, especially organ meats (liver, sweetbreads, tripe), shellfish, strong cheeses, and port wine ("rich men's food") should be avoided since they contain uric acid precursors. Gout is, in a way, a medically delightful disease if there is such a thing! It is, unlike most of the other arthritic diseases, almost always dramatically diagnosable, curable, and preventable.

Sports Injuries

Activities, sporting or otherwise, which require vigorous use of the upper extremities may result in problems with the elbow and shoulder. For instance, tennis elbow, marked by painful movement and occasional swollen tenderness of that joint, usually means a bursitis or tendonitis of the tendons of the forearm muscles. Tendonitis of the shoulder, also a form of bursitis, is associated with the inability to raise the arm and tendons over the front and side of the upper arm. In these cases the tendons and their associated sheaths (bursae) are frayed and inflamed. Treatment consists of rest of the affected joints by splinting and/or a sling, the use of an anti-inflammatory medicine (aspirin, ibuprofen) orally, or a cortisone injection into the inflamed area by your doctor. Physical therapy such as heat, gentle range of motion exercise, and massage with or without liniments, may also be helpful.

Knee injuries, particularly those associated with sports such as track events, basketball, and football where stressful rotation or twisting of the knee is frequent, have become commonplace and have given rise to a busy new subspecialty of orthopedics—knee surgery. The delicate internal ligaments (the cruciate ligaments) and cartilages are easily torn. Although they may heal spontaneously if only partially torn and good conservative care is provided, more often, in my experience, surgery (usually arthroscopic) may be necessary for repair. It usually is successful.

A general rule about musculoskeletal injuries: An injured structure, even when healed by nature or surgery, may never again be as good as new and, therefore, the injured person needs to be particularly wary and protective of reinjury, even if it means giving up the activity that caused it. This can be a bitter pill to swallow; just ask Sandy Koufax or Bo Jackson.

Vigorous bodily activity, sports and athletics included, is prone to cause accidents by its very nature. Sports or not, injuries are injuries. The principal distinction is that if you are a professional athlete or the injury occurs on the job, then the costs, at least, are usually covered by either your contract or workers' compensation. The type of injury (fracture, sprain, strain) is determined by the activity that produced it. For instance, sports that involve jumping, jogging, or otherwise pounding the axial skeleton and weight-bearing joints tend to cause either sprains, strains, or stress (pressure) fractures of the structures that take the beating. Activities involving twisting or turning forcefully, thereby stressing ligaments and tendons holding joints and bones in place, invariably tear these structures when they are overtaxed. In fact, sports such as football, hockey, and boxing combine the above forces with actual crushing-type pressure to the body parts exposed. From the medical viewpoint the martial arts, which have their advantages and their devoted adherents, may not be good for the health and well-being of the players unless, by virtue of their mastery, they are able to avoid violence. This is, according to the true experts, the reason for their being in the first place.

DR. DASHE'S TIPS FOR HEALTH MAINTENANCE

1. A rudimentary knowledge of your anatomy will help in the maintenance of your bones and muscles.

2. Prevention is much better than treatment. Using your knowledge of anatomy and the types of injuries and ailments will help avoid placing your muscles or bones at risk.

3. Just because your feet are farthest from your head doesn't diminish their importance. Proper maintenance and comfortable footwear can help ensure lifelong mobility.

4. Before exercising it is important that you properly stretch leg muscles. This will help avoid cramping and shin splints.

5. The knee is by far the most susceptible and traumatic area for sports injury. Beyond abstinence, prevention is difficult; a modicum of care may put the odds in your favor.

6. Back problems are ubiquitous and incapacitating because of the upright stature of man. Back care, including postural exercises, before or after back trouble, is necessary to remain comfortable vertically. The neck is another susceptible area of the spine for similar reasons.

7. There are a number of noninvasive remedies available to relieve back pain; make surgery your last resort.

8. Osteoporosis is a relatively rare occurence in men so calcium supplementation, unless ordered by your doctor, is not usually necessary in an otherwise healthy diet.

9. Osteoarthritis in men occurs most often in the knees and hips. The best way to deal with this common affliction is to stay active and get exercise; swimming especially is beneficial.

10. As always moderation in your activity is to your ultimate benefit. Too much exercise can lead to traumatic injury and breakdown of cartilage. So, "Just do it," but not too much.

Chapter 6

THE HEART AND CARDIOVASCULAR SYSTEM

By now you have noted that the tone of this book tends toward reassurance based on the favorable trends in American health statistics. Indeed, if deaths from violence and AIDS are removed from the statistics, the prognosis for American males has never been so good. This has in no small part been accomplished by advances in our knowledge of the causation, treatment, and most importantly, prevention of serious diseases of the heart and blood vessels (cardiovascular system). As recently as thirty years ago, there was great debate as to whether high blood pressure was even a disease! It is. We knew little of the mechanism and causes of heart attack, much less how to treat it. We are now surely out of the dark ages, though we are just beginning to understand the whys and wherefores of cardiovascular disease. We shall discuss what is known and what is not, and what is in between. Some definitions will help you comprehend the information.

Heart

The heart is the incredible, indefatigable pump that lies in the middle of our chest, bulging to the left a bit that, for all our lives, night and day, through thick and thin, war and peace, keeps pumping away, keeping us in oxygen and nutrients for life (Figure 6-1).

This is a four-chambered, four-valve structure which actually pumps two circulations, the pulmonary and systemic. The pulmonary (lung) circulation involves the right chambers and valves, taking spent, deoxygenated blood from our

---

Figure 6-1: THE HEART

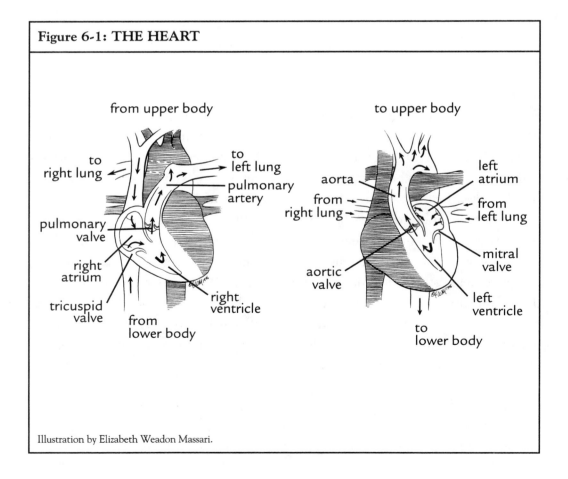

Illustration by Elizabeth Weadon Massari.

main veins (vena cavae) and sending it through the lungs to reoxygenate. The left side of the heart receives the freshly oxygenated blood from the lungs via the pulmonary veins. Utilizing its main muscle, the left ventricle, it then sends the fresh blood through the aortic valve into the aorta (main artery of the body) from whence it is distributed throughout the body. This is called the systemic circulation. The heart itself receives the first shot of fresh blood through the coronary ("crownlike") arteries which have their openings at the very base of the aorta. These obviously are vital tubes, for the heart needs a constant supply of fresh oxygen to do its mighty work. Interruption is disaster!

Vascular (Circulatory) System

Arteries

These are the thick-walled muscular, elastic tubes that conduct oxygen-rich blood from the heart and, in a treelike fashion, to the areas of the body served (Figure 6-2). They are deeply placed and cannot be seen from outside the body (except in the retina). They may be felt as pulsations, however, in many areas of the body, especially the thumb side of the wrist, the neck, and the groin (the "pulse points"). The pulsations occur when the heart pumps blood into the aorta and, therefore, when timed, accurately reflect the rate of the heartbeat. The elastic artery wall actually dampens the shock of the forceful injection of blood into the aorta. These pulsations create sounds (called Korotkov sounds) which may be heard via a stethoscope while utilizing a blood pressure cuff (sphygmomanometer). These sounds are used in determining the pressure of the blood in the artery. Such blood pressure devices are now commonly used by laypersons who wish to determine this information for themselves or for guidance in the treatment of high blood pressure (hypertension—see page 89). The arteries branch down into smaller and smaller tubules (arterioles) until they are small enough to service the tiniest blood vessels of them all, the capillaries.

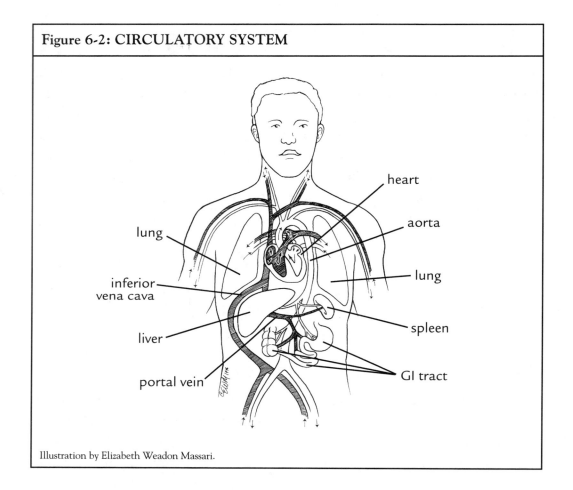

Figure 6-2: CIRCULATORY SYSTEM

Illustration by Elizabeth Weadon Massari.

Capillaries

These slim, delicate tubules are too tiny to be seen with the naked eye. Indeed, they are just wide enough to permit passage of one or two blood corpuscles at a time. They supply all of our living tissues and provide the transfer of oxygen and fuel to the tissues at the first part of the capillary. The end of the capillary is where used fuel and carbon dioxide from metabolized oxygen is picked up and returned to the larger vessels known as venules, which are the beginning of the venous (vein) system.

Veins

These are thin-walled, nonpulsing vessels that take up the "used" blood into ever-enlarging branches which eventually end in the main veins, the upper and lower (superior and inferior) vena cavae. They have no muscle or elasticity and, therefore, require actual valves to keep blood going in the right direction (heart-ward) and not down to the legs by the force of gravity. The venous blood is much darker than the freshly oxygenated kind and, therefore, appears, when seen through the skin, as blue-colored cords. The veins tend to be quite superficial and are easily seen in the extremities, especially when the extremity is held below the heart level, as when standing with arms dangling. Venous blood ends up in the vena cavae and then back to the heart for reprocessing. Pressure in the veins, therefore, is nil when one is horizontal. All veins tend to collapse or decrease in diameter unless there is obstruction to the flow back to the heart.

Arteriosclerosis

This literally means hardening of the arteries, and is usually caused by the deposition of cholesterol salts and calcium into the walls of the vessels. Atherosclerosis is the proper medical term but these words are used interchangeably.

Hypertension

It means elevation of blood pressure above normal as determined by direct or indirect measurement using a sphygmomanometer. The measurements are defined as millimeters (mm) of mercury, as in a barometer. The definition of normal range may vary with the authority consulted but the consensus currently is that the normal resting blood pressure should not exceed 140 mm/90 mm of mercury. The upper, or systolic, number refers to the pressure at the time of maximum heart pumping (contraction of the heart). The lower, or diastolic, number is the pressure in the vessels with the heart at rest between beats. The diastolic is actually the basic pressure at all times and, therefore, most important in the determination if one is hypertensive.

Recent research has shown that elevation of systolic blood pressure is also of importance. Systolic hypertension with a normal or low diastolic pressure, if transient, had traditionally been of little concern and simply considered a reaction to harder pumping caused by physical or emotional exertion. Persistent systolic elevation was seen to be a function of the aging process with the accompanying stiffness of the major arteries. A large study of an aging population, recently completed, showed that lowering of systolic high blood pressure significantly improved health and decreased the incidence of severe cardiovascular disease. It is now current practice to treat systolic hypertension (over 150 mm of mercury) with appropriate antihypertensive medicines.

Incidentally, life insurance actuarial tables, upon which life insurance premiums are based, are heavily weighted toward blood pressure measurements. These business-oriented folks are not only interested in your health. They are betting money on your longevity, so their tables are likely to be accurate.

Diseases of the Cardiovascular System

Arteriosclerosis

Arteriosclerosis is by far the most frequent cause of death in the American male (females too, as a matter of fact). It is a process that leads to narrowing and closure of the vital vessels that supply our organs, particularly the heart, brain, and kidneys. If there is acute stoppage, such as when a rapid clot formation occurs, devastating, sudden, acute disease may occur such as in heart attack or stroke. Gradual narrowing, which is more common, is apt to cause more subtle, albeit ominous symptoms such as angina pectoris or transient visual disturbances. The causes of arteriosclerosis are many and there are a number of contributing factors.

Aging is the most obvious cause. The older artery, simply by wear and tear and exposure to normal pounding will, even under the best of circumstances, gradually harden. It has been found in incidental autopsies of young men ages fifteen to thirty that fatty streaks or other beginnings of arteriosclerosis may be present, indicating the necessity of starting preventive measures as early as possible, even in childhood (diet and exercise again, avoidance of fast-food fat overload).

Hypertension is a cardinal factor. The harder the pounding of the blood pressure on the arterial walls, the sooner they wear out. Control of hypertension, which is a relatively recent medical advance, probably accounts for much of the great improvement in statistics for the diseases associated with arteriosclerosis.

Biochemical causes—cholesterol, cholesterol, cholesterol. This material is a normal and vital chemical in our blood and is a metabolic precursor for many of our hormones and cellular structures. We could not live without it, so despite adverse media attention, it must not be abolished from the earth. Most of the body's cholesterol is not derived from ingested food but is rather manufactured by the liver from precursor fats, particularly the solid or saturated ones. Cholesterol is carried in blood attached to other, larger molecules known as lipoproteins, some of which are small and dense (high density) and some large and "fluffy" (low density). The latter kind, low-density lipoprotein cholesterol (LDL) is more easily pounded into the arterial walls. The high-density type (HDL) tends to remain dissolved and even seems somehow to protect the walls from this fatty coating. This is an oversimplification of a complex process; it is important to keep your HDL high and LDL low. This may not be easy, but if one is lucky enough to be born with the right genes (again, there is a strong genetic factor here), control of weight and appropriate dietary measures definitely help. A little red wine may be helpful (see French Paradox, pages 6–7). Triglycerides, another type of blood fat, consist of large molecules of fatty acids, mostly those absorbed from the fat digested in the intestinal tract attached to a glycerol molecule to form large particles known as chylomicrons. These large fat particles are carried to the liver for metabolic conversion and used in various ways. High levels of triglycerides in the blood appear after eating a high-fat-containing meal and take time (up to twelve hours) to be cleared from the bloodstream. There are genetic disorders, called hyperlipidemias, that are associated with premature and severe arteriosclerosis, among other problems (skin lesions and pancreatitis), but the most common disorder associated with high triglycerides is Type 2 diabetes. In any case, triglyceride levels, which must be checked when you are fasting, are now considered to be important indications, if not a direct cause of arteriosclerosis.

Other causes of arteriosclerosis include diabetes, obesity, hypothyroidism, familial metabolic disorders, and especially tobacco smoking (the mechanism for this is unknown at the present time). There is much argument whether exercise by itself is a helpful factor, other than helping to keep one's weight down.

In any case, once cholesterol is established and embedded in the wall of the artery, a destructive process commences. There is actual erosion and even ulceration, resulting in fibrous scarring and deposition of calcium into the damaged area. These raw areas are subject to clot formation, usually when blood platelets adhere and start a cascade of clotting events. This is a natural healing response to injury, but represents an over-response that is dangerous. Whether or not clotting happens, the artery is damaged, usually narrowed, and the blood supply is curtailed. Sometimes the wall of the artery may be so damaged that the pressure of the blood may thin it out and cause an abnormal bulge, known as an aneurysm. All of these events are bad news for the body.

Coronary Thrombosis

Occlusion, heart attack, coronary, or myocardial infarction due to coronary artery arteriosclerosis are all names for the same condition. This refers to the devastating and potentially fatal situation caused by acute blockage of one of the coronary arteries. These vessels provide the blood supply to the heart muscle itself. There are three main arteries, which vary in size. The most important is usually the front one, called the left anterior descending coronary artery. The right coronary and circumflex coronary arteries are usually of somewhat lesser import, since they generally supply less vital areas of heart muscle. The left anterior descending artery supplies the left ventricle, the largest and most vital pump chamber. The left anterior descending artery was given the dubious honor of being labeled the "artery of sudden death" and "widow maker." Sudden blockage of this artery by clot is often found on postmortem examination and is thought to be the most frequent cause of that sudden, dramatic demise, the fatal heart attack. Fortunately, we now know a lot more about causes, symptoms, treatment, and prevention of this deadly process. Almost all of this has been learned in the past forty years.

Now that we have reviewed the cause, let's discuss the symptoms and treatment of this arteriosclerotic catastrophe.

Symptoms and Treatment of Heart Attack

The heart, being a muscle, may, as do all of our muscles, manifest distress with the symptom of cramping pain. This pain, caused by deprivation of oxygen to the hard-working heart muscle, is perceived in areas supplied by nerves that also serve the neck and chest and upper extremities. Cardiac pain, therefore, was given the old name of angina (Latin meaning "pain in the throat") or angina pectoris (pectoris = chest). The pain is generally a constricting, cramping discomfort which may occur almost anyplace between the jaw and the diaphragm. It generally starts mildly and increases with time, usually in minutes. The pain is frequently associated with sweating and/or nausea and, in some cases, an impending feeling of doom. It is usually constant and unremitting, although sometimes it comes and goes before it finally persists and aid is sought. I cannot emphasize enough that immediate emergency aid is warranted in such circumstances. Time is of the greatest importance. If the patient can get to an emergency room within the first hour or two of the onset of pain, clot-dissolving drugs may be administered and heart muscle damage completely avoided. This is a modern medical miracle. (Incidentally, it seems that taking an aspirin immediately may be helpful as an emergency anticoagulant clot dissolver.) Even if clot dissolving cannot be accomplished, it is now possible, by doing emergency coronary angiography (x-ray-guided cardiac catheterization and visualization of the arteries—moving pictures of the vessels and the blood flowing through them) to possibly stretch open the narrowed or clotted artery with a special balloon tube (angioplasty). Current practice now includes the use of permanent metal expanders (stents), which may be fitted by catheter into the stretched vessel to keep it from closing down again. These stents are getting better and better in design and performance and may replace many more invasive measures. If this is not possible, more radical procedures are still available to save the heart muscle and the victim's life. Coronary artery bypass surgery (with vein or artery grafts placed between the aorta and the unblocked portions of the coronary artery) is now as commonplace as appendectomy. Again, success is dependent upon *rapid* action.

Pericarditis

This condition, associated with similar severe chest pains, is due to acute inflammation of the pericardial membranes (or sac) that surround the heart. Usually caused by an infection (almost always viral), it is rarely fatal and is treatable with various nonradical measures. The trick is diagnosis, which is not difficult to make for an experienced internist or cardiologist. It is rarely life threatening. I have discussed this further in the section "Pulmonary Pain" on page 96.

Noncardiac Chest Pains

I have previously mentioned the frantic phone calls received by doctors from patients who think they are having a heart attack. Fortunately, the home diagnosis is usually incorrect, sincere as the patient may be. This is because pain in the left side of the chest is usually equated with heart pain. It is more often due to something else; often digestive problems. Gastrointestinal pain is not infrequently experienced in the chest, whereas cardiac pain is almost never felt in the abdomen.

Gastrointestinal Pains in the Chest

Esophageal pain. The esophagus, or swallowing tube, descends from the throat down to the stomach. Plainly, it must pass through the chest, and its route is a strategic one. It passes directly behind the heart itself on its way through the opening (called the hiatus) in the diaphragm where it empties into the stomach. The lower end of this structure is a muscular valve known as the lower esophageal sphincter which, when closed, prevents regurgitation of stomach contents back into the esophagus. The esophagus itself is a muscular tube (see pages 151, 154–155) which contracts rhythmically to push swallowed material into the stomach. It's very strong—it is even possible to swallow liquids or solids standing on your head, if you are curious enough to try such a maneuver. Its muscular contractions can be powerful and even painful at times. Such pain will be perceived, frequently with alarm, deep in the midchest; it can be sudden, sharp, and seems to be the heart for sure. Heart pain, on the other hand, is almost always slow in onset and dull, building gradually to a climax. Esophageal muscle spasm may be caused by many things, including heat or cold, irritation of any sort, or most commonly, emotional stress. It will generally subside by itself, but often simply swallowing a sip of water will make it go away. In any case, the act of swallowing will modify the discomfort enough to usually suggest the diagnosis of noncardiac esophagus pain.

Other common esophageal pain, such as that associated with dyspepsia (see page 159) may respond rapidly to an antacid such as Maalox or Mylanta. Dyspeptic pain is usually a burning sensation in the low midchest, hence the term "heartburn," which, literally speaking, it isn't; it has nothing to do with the heart.

More serious and of greater concern is chronic gastroesophageal regurgitation (or GERD, see pages 154–155), which usually is manifested by chronic recurrent heartburn, particularly after eating or when reclining. Management of this problem is described in the section on gastrointestinal disorders.

Gallbladder pain. Inflammation of the gallbladder, usually associated with gallstones (see page 161) may be confused with heart pain. Usually felt in the shoulder blade area, it may also cause low-front chest pain and upper mid-abdominal pain.

Gas pain in the colon. A common, frightening left-sided chest pain may be caused by a bit of trapped gas in the part of the left colon situated right beneath the left diaphragm. This area, known as the splenic flexure, is part of the large bowel that makes a sharp bend as it crosses the abdominal cavity from right to left and then descends downward to the rectum (Figure 10-1, page 151). When a large bubble gets trapped there, the colon, which at that point is actually fairly high up in the chest, may spasm in response to the gassy distention. One will feel a sharp, crampy pain around the left breast prompting, on occasion, a 911 call. Treatment consists of relaxation, if possible, and cessation of gum chewing and nervous gulping, which is a major cause of air swallowing and subsequent increased bowel gas. Various simethicone preparations (GasX®, Mylicon®) are touted for chronic recurrence of this embarassing condition. These may or may not help, but are worth trying.

Pulmonary Pain

The bronchial tubes and the lungs do register pain when troubled and irritated by fumes such as smoke and smog. Bronchial infections and pneumonias are potentially painful, particularly when severe and acute and associated with coughing. Because of the associated symptoms of cough, fever, and expectoration, the question of heart attack usually doesn't arise. One dire situation, however, is that of pulmonary embolism. This usually is caused by a clot that has broken off from a clotted vein from the legs or pelvis and then travels to the lungs, producing sudden, severe pain anyplace in the chest. This clotting typically occurs after injury or surgery or, on occasion, after a long airplane trip when the legs are kept in one cramped position. (Remember to get up and walk around or at least stretch your legs!) It calls for medical testing for the proper diagnosis, which is not at all easy unless the doctor thinks of it.

Pleurisy is pain due to inflammation of the membranes surrounding the lungs, the pleura. If these are inflamed from any cause, pain will result. This can be brought on by chest movement during breathing, a diagnostic tip-off. Heart pain is not brought on by taking a breath. Pleurisy may be caused by infection or inflammation from any cause, frequently a transient but painful virus. Epidemic viral pleurisy was first named after places that had such epidemics: Coxsackie (New Jersey) disease, Bornholm (Island) disease, or a more dramatic appellation, "Devils Grip." Pleurisy is very painful with the chest movement of breathing or coughing, but clearly it is not heart disease because of the nature of the pain.

More difficult to distinguish but related to pleurisy is pericarditis, which is a painful inflammation of the wrapping membranes (the pericardium) of the heart. Not only does this cause constant pain, since the heart is always in motion, but it may cause some confusing abnormalities of the electrocardiogram. A doctor is able to distinguish this, usually without difficulty, from a more serious disease of the heart muscle itself. Treatment with anti-inflammatory medicines usually produces dramatic relief.

Pneumothorax

Finally, severe, sudden chest pain, usually unilateral (right or left) may be caused by a small rupture of the lung wrapping (pleural membrane), which permits escape of air into that side of the chest cavity. This is called pneumothorax. This happens, not infrequently, in response to some traumatic event (e.g., stabbing, blow to the chest, violent exercise). Sometimes, however, it can be quite spontaneous. The lung collapse, fortunately, is usually partial and one-sided so that breathing is maintained. Treatment consists of watchful waiting for spontaneous healing and air absorption (if the free air is a small amount and the hole in the pleural membrane is small). Or frequently, the placement of a small suction tube between the ribs is performed, which re-expands the lung and permits healing to take place, usually in a day or two. It is possible to make a phone diagnosis of this condition, if the situation is a "set up" for its occurrence. Prompt diagnosis and treatment is advisable.

Chest Pain Due to Chest Wall Troubles

The chest is a more or less rigid cage composed of bone (the thoracic spine, the ribs, and the breastbone, or sternum), movable joints composed of cartilage to bone connections, and muscle. All of these structures are potential sources of pain. The chest wall muscles, between the ribs, are used in respiratory movements. These muscles are subject, as are any muscles, to sprain (for example, with an athletic injury or even a hard or persistent cough). The pain is usually pleuritic in nature; that is, aggravated by breathing, but may be constant, a source of great consternation. It is harmless, though, and amenable to the simple measures used to treat any other muscle ache—heat, rest, analgesics, and/or anti-inflammatory medicines. The joints of ribs to breastbone, cartilaginous in nature, are called costo-chondral joints (costo = rib, chondro = cartilage) and are subject to a kind of arthritis known as costochondritis. This may cause a chronic pain and tenderness over the front of the chest that is mistaken for heart pain. The tip-off is the presence of tenderness directly over the painful area. Chest wall pain in general is marked by soreness and tenderness and aggravation by movement, especially coughing and sneezing. Pain is relieved by analgesics and judicious splinting of the chest wall by use of a wide, soft belt across the lower rib cage. Immobilizing the lower ribs prevents motion of the entire chest. Commercial Velcro® fastened rib belts are useful, since these splints should be removed frequently to permit full lung and chest expansion from time to time. I recall my own experience with some painful broken ribs. Coughing and sneezing were hellish experiences, but I discovered that jamming my chest up against a doorway provided enough splinting for comfort at such times.

In any event, these noncardiac pains eventually go away.

Angina Without Heart Attack

I have emphasized, with reason, the worst possible scenario for the illness caused by arteriosclerosis of the coronary arteries—that is, coronary thrombosis. The purpose is simply to alert one to the danger and the necessity for immediate response. A far more common situation, however, is the condition known simply as angina, which I have already described as a symptom, rather than a disease. Arteriosclerotic heart disease is the actual primary disorder. The causal mechanism is the narrowing of the coronary vessel so that the blood flow is restricted to some degree. Occasionally, the effect can be caused by spastic narrowing of the coronary artery with or without arteriosclerotic change. Nitroglycerine and other medicines, which are used in this condition, alleviate this spastic narrowing by relaxing the vessel. Angina is frequently asymptomatic until the point is reached where the heart muscle cannot get enough oxygenated blood to meet its energy requirement. The harder and faster the heart must pump (directly proportional to the load placed upon it by exertion, physical or emotional), the greater the oxygen requirement. The previously described pain may, therefore, occur at such times of exertion. Angina actually may be manifested by symptoms other than pain. These include weakness, shortness of breath, and tingling or numbness of an upper extremity or almost any place between the face and the lower chest or upper back. Occasionally a palpitation, a skipped, irregular or rapid heartbeat, is perceived. The symptoms characteristically go away when the stress is relieved by rest or relaxation. But one's physician should promptly investigate anything resembling these symptoms. The diagnosis can be made, usually via noninvasive methods in the doctor's office or cardiology laboratory. A disastrous heart attack may be avoided by early detection and treatment. Angina syndrome may be ameliorated by various medications (nitroglycerin preparations, beta blocker drugs, and calcium channel blocker drugs). Aspirin therapy (see page 101) also is warranted if not otherwise contraindicated. More frequently nowadays angiography is being done early after initial diagnosis, since angioplasty and bypass procedures have become safer, more commonplace, and more routine. This is a somewhat controversial matter. Probably more of these invasive measures are done than are absolutely necessary since more and more cardiologists (activists mostly, in my experience) are oriented this way. Certainly some, if not the majority, of these patients will require such invasive intervention eventually and it is still difficult to determine which are which. There is no question, however, that many patients may get along quite nicely and live normal life spans with adequate medical measures and lifestyle changes (*stop smoking, lose excess weight, exercise moderately, take aspirin and other helpful medicines, get blood pressure down to normal range, get cholesterol under control with diet and, if necessary, take cholesterol-lowering medicine, and practice relaxation techniques*).

As far as diet is concerned, I have already discussed several of the controversial issues in previous chapters. There is little or no doubt, however, of the immense value of dietary lifestyle changes in cases of obesity or those with high-fat diets. Weight reduction will invariably tend to normalize the blood fat levels, particularly to lower the bad, LDL, and raise the good, HDL. Cutting the percentage of all fats, especially the saturated type (meats, dairy fats, tropical oils such as coconut) leads to the same beneficial change in HDL to LDL ratio, as does cutting total fats to less than 20 percent of total caloric intake (10 percent is even better). Only when these maneuvers have been tried, and the blood fat ratios remain unfavorable, are the cholesterol-lowering drugs appropriate. Dietetic advice is available widely, but if books and magazines are too contradictory or confusing, consultation with a reliable (preferably registered) dietician may be useful. Your doctor can refer you to one. My advice regarding nutrition specialists, M.D. or not, is generally to stay away. They tend to be faddish, expensive, and vitamin salespeople.

Exercise is another confusing and controversial matter. There is some evidence that regular exercise may improve established arteriosclerotic disease, but always in conjunction with other lifestyle adjustments, so it is truly impossible to ascribe definitive value to this modality. Cardiac rehabilitation clinics accentuate moderate, regular exercise as I have previously described. The secret is getting oneself to do this consistently. Perhaps, then, a structured exercise program may be the answer for some. I have found no convincing evidence that exercise alone will prolong life or cure the disease. Fanatic overexertion is dangerous and may be deadly.

Cholesterol-lowering drugs, such as niacin (nicotinic acid) and HMG-CoA reductase (liver enzyme) inhibitors such as lovastatin (Mevocor®) and others have received much favorable attention lately. Some experts feel strongly that the evidence points to real amelioration of arteriosclerosis with the use of these somewhat expensive medicines, combined with other lifestyle measures. Antioxidant supplements such as beta carotene and vitamins E and C are still controversial, although most studies indicate that a diet rich in these substances (lots of fruits, vegetables, and grains) is the answer. Some authorities still recommend vitamin E, 400 to 800 units per day, despite the controversies in evidence.

Certain classes of medication, namely the beta blockers, such as propranolol (Inderal®) and nadolol (Corgard®), and calcium channel blockers, such as diltiazem (Cardizem®) and amlodipine (Norvasc®), along with lowering blood pressure, may slow the arteriosclerotic process.

Finally, a word about "Syndrome X," which has become a fanciful term for what appears to be a very common cluster of bad things that happen to middle-aged people. These are abnormal elevations of blood pressure, mild hypertension, high levels of insulin in the blood ("resistance" with or without obvious diabetes Type 2), central obesity (midsection rather than hips and thighs), and high triglyceride (blood fats). People affected with this combination, according to experts such as Dr. Peter Pool of UC San Diego and Dr. William Castelli of the Framingham Project, will have coronary events. The only question is when. The happy news, if you want to call it that, is that this syndrome is very responsive to a strict diet and exercise program, with total reversibility an achievable goal. Medicines, including aspirin, antioxidants, and cholesterol-lowering drugs, are only adjunctive measures but are helpful. Castelli even suggests that asymptomatic people with this syndrome would benefit by going to a cardiac rehabilitation clinic before an attack, thus avoiding it altogether. A radical suggestion, interesting and not likely to happen, unfortunately, but at least the ideas are useful.

A word about aspirin. I was privileged, some fifteen years ago, to be included in the Physicians Health Study at Harvard Medical School in which 22,000 male doctors between the ages of forty and eighty-four were given 5 grains of aspirin or a placebo (phony pill) to take every other day. The researchers wanted to note the effect on cardiovascular disease. After five years we subjects received a rather complaining, cranky letter stating that we were all too healthy. Nobody died. The study, therefore, continued for another year. At the end of the sixth year we were notified that the research referee had intervened. The aspirin group had suffered significantly fewer heart attacks and, therefore, the conclusion, statistically at least, was that aspirin somehow protected against coronary thrombosis. (I was informed, incidentally, that I had been taking a placebo. Since I had not suffered a coronary thrombosis during this period, I was a little apprehensive to stop taking the placebo!) The mechanism whereby aspirin prevents clots seems to be via those little platelets, which plug up tiny holes in our blood vessel walls and start the clot process (the cascade). Aspirin, it seems, makes the platelets slightly less sticky and therefore prevents sudden clot formation, although it does not prevent the arteriosclerotic process. Subsequently it has been found to be helpful in other similar arteriosclerotic disorders such as artery hardening in the vessels to the brain and lower extremities. A small amount, even a children's aspirin (81 mg), does the trick. Aspirin (any type) every other day seems to be all that is needed. I continue to take this and advise my patients, male and female, to do the same, although the beneficial effect on the female has not yet been proven (studies are still underway). Some people, of course, cannot take aspirin for whatever reason; check with your doctor.

A word about cholesterol-lowering measures. It appears that lowering the LDL cholesterol and raising the HDL is protective against progressive arteriosclerotic changes (see pages 91–92). I have mentioned the dietary measures (more monounsaturated fat, less saturated fat, and less than 25 percent of either in one's daily diet), perhaps a small amount of red wine or other alcohol, and trimming obesity as much as possible. If all else fails, there are now medications that, if taken regularly and under professional guidance, are safe and effective agents to accomplish the job. These include niacin (a B vitamin) in large amounts and certain aforementioned liver enzyme blockers (for example, Mevacor) which prevent the conversion of saturated fats to cholesterol. There is still some controversy about how effective these somewhat expensive medicines are, but they appear to be safe enough, at least when used properly.

Hypertension

I have alluded to the "new" disease, hypertension, or high blood pressure. I remember, with some awe, reading the diary of Admiral (Dr.) Macyntyre, who took care of our former president, Franklin D. Roosevelt. President Roosevelt suffered from elevated blood pressure and indeed died prematurely at the age of sixty-four (a few months before World War II ended in 1945), from the worst complication of hypertension, a massive brain hemorrhage. His physician noted that the president's blood pressure was "very high," 240/160, and there was no help for it except to sedate Mr. Roosevelt with phenobarbital! There was simply no effective, specific medicine for elevated blood pressure, and none became available for another ten years. There was no consensus on the significance of elevated blood pressure until the 1960s, when it became clear, after many studies, that hypertension was indeed a disease—a deadly one at that.

The causes of hypertension are still not completely clear. It is known now that the majority of instances of hypertension are of unknown cause and are called "primary" (a euphemism for "we don't know"). Various theories of causation include environmental stresses (hypertension is rarely seen in low-key societies), high salt intake, and heredity, but no definite cause has been isolated unless you consider "Syndrome X" the culprit, as does Dr. Pool (see page 100).

Far less frequent is the so-called "secondary" variety. That is, blood pressure elevation due to a known other primary cause, such as abnormal hormonal stimulus from disease of the kidneys or adrenal glands, or constriction of the renal (kidney) artery or aorta.

Hypertension needs to be evaluated and treated, for if undetected and untreated it can be a silent, deadly killer. Elevated blood pressure rarely causes discomfort until the damage it causes manifests itself. More commonly the damage is to the heart and arteries. The elevated pressure is an excessive load upon the heart muscle, leading in some cases to heart muscle strain and enlargement. In the last stages heart failure may ensue, which is the inability of the heart to carry this load. There is backup of blood into the venous circulation of the lungs and body. Symptoms of shortness of breath and swelling of the lower extremities may result.

Of even greater importance is the previously mentioned effect of hypertension on the wall of the arteries, premature arteriosclerosis. Control of elevated blood pressure prevents this. It is felt that management of hypertension is in large part responsible for a marked decrease of cardiovascular death and disease in our population in the past three decades.

We now have a large variety of effective antihypertension medicines. These include entire classes of drugs such as diuretics, beta blockers, calcium channel blockers, ACE inhibitors, alpha neuronal blockers, and others. The choice of medicines must be individualized, and requires close cooperation with your doctor and compliance on the part of the patient. These drugs can have side effects that make them intolerable to some people. We now are usually able to find the right medicine, or combination, for everyone. The newer ACE-inhibitor group and the long-acting calcium channel blockers are particularly well tolerated by men. The other drugs tend to carry a high incidence of sexual dysfunction, but these don't.

Get your blood pressure checked!

DR. DASHE'S TIPS FOR HEALTH MAINTENANCE

1. Disease and mortality from cardiovascular disease have shown major declines in American men in the past three decades due to our recent understanding of causes and prevention.

2. Arteriosclerosis is still the major cause of death in United States, but you have the ability to decrease your chances by lowering your fat intake, taking cholesterol-reducing medications, and controlling diabetes and obesity.

3. Hypertension has been found to aggravate arteriosclerosis. It can be treated with lifestyle changes as well as medication.

4. Sudden chest or arm pain requires prompt emergency intervention; if a clot has formed in a narrowed artery (arteriosclerosis) lifesaving anti-clotting measures need to be taken ASAP.

5. Not every chest pain has to do with the heart, but the stakes are too high to rely on your guess work; let your doctor sort it out.

6. Narrowed coronary arteries may cause exertional chest or arm pain without heart attack. This is called angina and may be treated with a variety of measures including lifestyle modifications (diet and exercise), medications, and, if necessary, stretching or bypassing the affected vessels.

7. Once again, stress and tension can be a factor in increasing your chance of a heart attack. Find ways of relaxing and dealing with life on its terms and not always on your own.

8. Smoking and excessive drinking are conducive to heart disease. If you smoke you are also increasing the risk of heart disease in those who are exposed to your secondhand smoke, very likely someone close and dear to you. See the next chapter for more excellent reasons to quit this dangerous habit.

9. Prevention of heart disease is better than treatment. Early detection, especially of hypertension, is the key.

Chapter 7

THE RESPIRATORY SYSTEM

As I write this chapter, I am looking out over the (alleged) San Fernando Valley from the Santa Monica foothills to the beautiful rugged San Gabriel mountains some fifteen miles to the north of my home. The problem is I can't, at the moment, see either the Valley or the mountains because of the intervening grayish-brown haze that we Los Angeles denizens call smog. Yesterday, *The Los Angeles Times* reported that the air pollution problem has been much ameliorated in the past five years although "we still have a long way to go." It is not likely that the problem of air pollution will even be substantially mitigated as long as fossil fuels (oil, coal, natural gas) are burned as our energy source. Smog is a problem in most of our cities and highly populated areas. If we all move to Wyoming to rid ourselves of it, we will bring the enemy with us—with our cars.

What is this stuff that we are breathing doing to our lungs and bodies? The answer, at present, is that we don't really know, most of the time. Surely it cannot be good. Though sometimes it appears to be relatively harmless, the consensus is that it is at least irritating and at times life threatening or even deadly (for example, smog attacks in Donora, Pennsylvania, in 1948 and London, England, in 1952 had associated significant mortality).

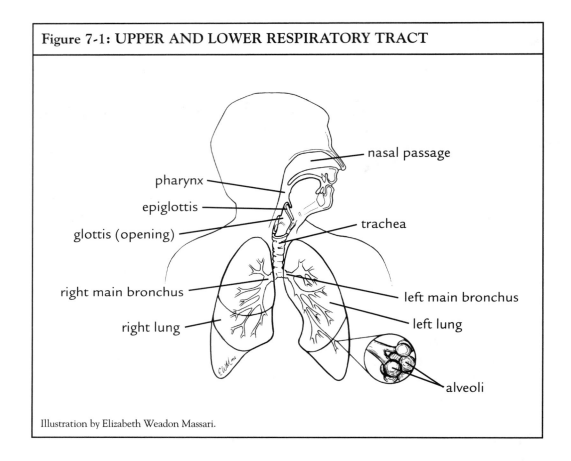

Figure 7-1: UPPER AND LOWER RESPIRATORY TRACT

Illustration by Elizabeth Weadon Massari.

The act of inspiring and then exhaling is known as respiration and this action takes place in the respiratory tract. The business of the respiratory system seems, on the face of it, simple. It is, but as with every other aspect of human design and function, it is a miraculous, neat, and beautiful piece of work (Figure 7-1).

The upper airway, consisting of the nasal passages and sinuses, filters (through a hairy network) and warms or cools, if necessary the inspired air, which then passes through the common channel for swallowing and breathing known as the pharynx. The glottis and the epiglottis flap function to shut off the air channels when we swallow liquid or solids. This vital action is both critical and automatic. Without it, we would literally drown or choke each time we swallowed fluid or food. As it is, we cough mightily when we swallow "the wrong way," meaning a speck of something other than air managed to get through the gate of the glottis. This cough, which forcefully expels air and foreign substances from the airway, is a powerful defense mechanism. The measured force of a normal cough is twenty to forty times the force used to simply exhale. The cough reflex is initiated simply by the irritation of the nerves supplying the back of the throat (posterior pharynx), the glottis, and the tracheo-bronchial surface membranes. To lose this reflex can mean death. (This is a devastating complication of some serious diseases of the central nervous system.) After air passes through the glottis, it goes to the trachea, the main breathing tube. This is a semirigid tube with ribs of cartilage that keep it from collapsing with the variable extremes of air pressure occurring during the breathing process. A smooth muscle underlies the delicate surface membrane. About 5 inches from its beginning the trachea divides into right and left branches known as the right and left main bronchi or bronchial tubes. The tracheal membrane and underlying muscle layer continue down into these main tubes and all the way down the branching tree known as the smaller branch bronchi. The smallest bronchi end in the tiny balloonlike cul-de-sacs known as alveoli—the place of oxygen absorption and carbon dioxide elimination.

The lungs, which consist of five lobes, three on the right side and two on the left, are tidy compartments for the alveoli. Each lobe is served by a subsidiary lobar bronchus. The entire tracheobronchial tree is lined with a special membrane, which has the capacity to secrete a viscous substance. This is called mucus and has the ability to capture foreign particles and noxious substances. These substances may then be expelled either by coughing or automatically via the cilia. These are little moving hairlets which are constantly picking up and pushing the mucus toward the glottis and thence to the pharynx, where it is usually swallowed and rendered innocuous. If the mucus is very abundant, it triggers a cough reflex and is then expelled via that route. Respiratory tract mucus is generally very thin, liquid, and colorless. However, during infection or fever with dehydration, mucus may become thick, colored, and hard to raise. The muscle fiber layers beneath the mucous membrane are important in the disease known as asthma.

As previously mentioned, the smallest bronchial branches, known as the terminal bronchi, finally end in tiny air sacs known as alveoli of the lungs. These minuscule chambers are made up of special cells one cell deep and are richly supplied with blood capillaries which, you will remember, are tiny tubules conducting only one or two red blood corpuscles at a time through their tiny diameters. These pulmonary capillaries are the site of a marvelous exchange of waste gas (carbon dioxide) released from the blood. This carbon dioxide is traded for a molecule of oxygen from the fresh air in the alveolus. The oxygen then attaches to the hemoglobin in the red blood cell.

Automatic timers in the brain drive respiration. These timers are in the respiratory centers of the medullary portion of the brain; a very primitive, automatic mechanism. That's why we don't have to remember to breathe when we sleep or are otherwise distracted. The neurons of the medullary part of the brain transmit signals down to the muscles of the diaphragm and the chest wall which cause the rhythmic contraction and relaxation that act as a bellows to pull air in and then expel it.

Common Diseases of
the Respiratory System

Snoring

This is a relative of sighing, yawning, and hiccuping. All are poorly understood modifications of the respiratory movement. The adaptive significance, biologically speaking, is even less clear. We men are supposed to be the greatest offenders but no one has ever studied the gender incidence of this supposedly unladylike night music. My wife snores and sounds like a buzz saw at times, and I, until a few years ago, thought myself free of such rude emissions. That is until I had occasion to share a hotel room with a colleague, who disappeared from the premises by the time of my awakening in the morning. He had changed his room in the middle of the night because, he said, of the infernal racket emanating from my bed. "But," I insisted, "I don't snore. My wife would have said something after all these years." "You have a marriage made in heaven!" was his response.

Here is controversy again. Is snoring a disease? Sleep clinics exist that provide help for this ancient plague. The question is not simply nose noise, but does this nocturnal pandemonium perhaps signify a fatal condition? I refer to sleep apnea syndrome which, according to some newspapers, is a major contributor to the obituary columns. This disorder is marked by cycles of snoring, then apparent choking, then seemingly interminable silence, followed by gasping. The cycles may repeat ad infinitum and have been likened to the potential equivalent of adult crib death. In my practice of internal medicine, I have heard many spousal descriptions of this phenomenon, but I never personally saw a fatal case. They have been reported nonetheless, and sleep monitoring has shown evidence of oxygen deprivation in severe cases. Nasal airway obstruction does, indeed, interfere with rest for some individuals, who may suffer from severe fatigue and sleepiness the following day.

I don't consider snoring a trivial matter. It is a real problem for snorer and listener. The problem may take a peculiar form. There was a famous letter to the editor of the *New England Journal of Medicine* a few years back in which a physician described a male patient with a mysterious pain in his right leg. It was severe and unresponsive to treatment and undiagnosed, despite x-rays, MRI scans, and many laboratory tests. Until one fateful night, when the man was awakened by a severe exacerbation of the sharp pain in his leg. He realized that he had been kicked by his wife. He whined "Why, oh why, did you kick me in my bad leg?" She answered, "I always kick you there when you snore." Diagnosis made. Case closed.

What, then, can be done about it? My advice to those most concerned is, first, relax. The danger is not so great. Then, it depends upon how bad the situation is. If the problem is mainly in the ear of the beholder, simple earplugs may suffice (the spongy plastic foam type work fine for me). If the snorer himself is truly bothered, more serious investigation and/or treatment may be in order. Although snoring usually is an entirely harmless process, it is often an indicator of some respiratory obstruction. The sound itself is produced by the flapping of the soft tissue of the pharynx (back of the throat) and, in the worst cases, the back of the tongue. Usually this occurs when the snorer is supine, face up, and is deeply asleep. The mouth is usually open. Nasal blockage problems such as allergies or colds may be prominent, and obesity is frequently associated with it. External nasal dilators (Breathe Right®), external or internal mucous membrane shrinkers (e.g., Afrin), may help but generally not much. Weight reduction may be extremely helpful. Surgery has become popular, especially laser-blasted holes through the soft palate tissues of the pharynx. All surgical methods are basically a "roto-rootering" of the pharyngeal airway. Surgical results vary, but probably are not better than fifty-fifty in most cases.

Before doing anything so extreme, I advise investigation by a legitimate sleep clinic or a specialist in pulmonary medicine. A simple device that is attached to the hand may be useful in screening for the dangerous forms of snoring. This pulse oximeter, as it's called, measures and records the amount of oxygen in the blood during the night, without actually touching the blood itself. It does so by shining a bright light through the tissues. If the study shows a normal amount of oxygen, usually this rules out the necessity for more complicated monitoring. This involves monitoring the patient throughout the night with instruments measuring respiration and heart action to see if truly significant obstruction is happening. This may be done in a sleep laboratory or at home. If necessary, various measures, including the more radical one of surgery, may be prescribed. There are some (still experimental) medications that may help and there is a mode of respiratory assistance used during the night known as a Continuous Positive Air Pressure device (C-PAP). It is a mask that fits over the nose of the patient and helps prevent oxygen deprivation by softly distending the flaccid pharynx and gently forcing air into the lungs. The C-PAP device is bothersome to many people but if used properly, it does cure the affliction most of the time. Major reconstructive surgery of the pharynx and neck is rarely indicated, but if done should be performed by an experienced surgical team, such as the one at Stanford University Hospital, which specializes in this procedure.

Upper Respiratory Infections

Common Cold. By far the most common incapacitating problem is the common cold (coryza); a miserable nonfatal malady, to be sure. These nasty afflictions are usually caused by a variety (rather than one) of viruses. If only one virus was responsible, I do not doubt that someone would have long since invented a trillion-dollar vaccine. The common cold is manifested by irritation (sneezing, coughing, runny nose, and increased mucus) of the nasopharyngeal and bracheobronchial membranes, as well as a general febrile malaise due to the invasion of the entire body by this pesky virus. Fortunately, viral colds go away in three to seven days. Sometimes, however, the swollen, battered membranes are invaded by opportunistic germs that are always hanging around, waiting for a chance to invade. These are the bacteria of various types (including streptococci, pneumonia organisms, and others). They will, if established enough, cause what are commonly called secondary infections, leading to what are known as bacterial pharyngitis (strep throat), sinusitis, bronchitis, and less often in the adult, otitis media (middle-ear infection). The secondary bacterial infections tend to be more violent and fever causing. They are also frequently associated with pus formation (collections of our disease-fighting white blood cells) in the affected areas—sinuses, pharynx and tonsils, and bronchial tubes. Hence the specific names—sinusitis, tonsillitis, pharyngitis, bronchitis. These problems are in the upper respiratory tract. Less commonly, when our upper defenses fail, the lungs themselves are involved, causing the much more serious disease pneumonia (in the lower respiratory tract). Pneumonias are more serious because of the involvement of the alveoli. Bacteria may gain entrance to the bloodstream through the alveolar capillary and cut off the vital oxygen absorption process.

Treatment of a Cold. The progression from a cold to pneumonia is a rare event. Paradoxically, pneumonia is still easier to cure than a cold! The reason is that we have no antibiotics for cold viruses but the bacteria that cause pneumonia are, for the most part, susceptible to these wonder drugs. We worry about the future because too often such drugs are wrongly and prematurely prescribed for viral illnesses. This leads to resistance to antibiotics by the bacterial invaders that may come later. It is simply too easy to prescribe these drugs for trivial infections, especially when the patient insists. The good medicine I have previously outlined (see pages 52–53) bears repetition: fluids, especially hot and spicy ones (broth, tea), rest, analgesics such as acetaminophen (Tylenol) or aspirin for fever and achiness. Decongestants, such as pseudoephedrine or phenylephrine, may give some relief from nasal congestion. Nasal sprays, such as Afrin (oxymetazoline) may be used judiciously; not more than one or two times per day because they can be addicting. Antihistamines are useless here. Cough medicines, usually containing guiafenesin and dextromethorphan, may help a bit, but stronger cough suppressants contain codeine or hydrocodone (e.g., Tussionex®) and require a prescription. (An interesting historical note: heroin, 5 mg tablets, was prescribed for colds by British doctors until a few decades ago.) If, however, a respiratory infection lasts more than three to four days, particularly with development of fever or yellow-green secretions from the nose or coughed up from the throat, bacterial infection is likely and first-line antibiotics are usually helpful in stemming it. It is to be noted that prior to the antibiotic era, people survived upper respiratory infections, though it took a bit longer.

Bronchitis

Inflammation and infection of the bronchial tubes may be acute or chronic. The acute type usually is secondary to a viral infection, which may then be complicated by a bacterial infection. The chronic type is far more serious, for it means that there is usually permanent damage to the bronchial membrane with loss of cilia function and recurrent secondary invasion by opportunistic bacteria. By far the most common cause of this miserable situation is chronic inflammation due to constant irritation from smoking. Other causes include air pollution in severely affected areas, allergies to various pollens or other particulates (dusts), or recurrent infections. Finally, there are some relatively rare hereditary diseases associated with bronchitis.

Chronic bronchitis is a serious medical problem and may lead to respiratory disability and even death, if not adequately managed. Bronchiectasis is a form of bronchitis in which pus-filled pockets in the bronchial tree may form, eventually causing chronic infection which is difficult to treat.

Pneumonia

As stated above, this is a serious infectious disease of the lower respiratory tract. Pneumonia due to the pneumococcus germ (Streptococcus pneumoniae is the scientific name) was, before the antibiotic era, the major cause of death in the American population, along with pulmonary tuberculosis (actually another form of more chronic pneumonia). Penicillin ended that for a time, but the pneumo-coccus is still around and still a serious hazard, particularly since antibiotic-resistant strains have evolved. A pneumococcal vaccine, which is *very effective*, is now available and is advisable for all adults.

The many other pneumonia-causing bugs range from funguses such as the one causing valley fever (coccidioidomycosis) to strange new ones like Le-gionella, the cause of Legionnaire's disease. This notorious epidemic, a mysteri-ous Agatha Christie-like event, sprung from a "new" bacteria sprayed on an American Legion convention via a contaminated air-conditioning unit. It was important for several reasons. First, it demonstrated that new invaders are com-ing up unexpectedly. Second, modern conveniences frequently may be the source of our downfall. Actually, this is nothing new; historically, it has always been thus. Syphilis was brought to the Old World from the New World via Columbus's vessels. AIDS was brought from Africa via the jet plane.

Pneumonias of all kinds are diagnosed by chest x-rays showing an area that is opaque (an infiltrate) in a previously clear area which should, on x-ray, look translucent. The symptoms range from mild (like a bad cold) to devastating (with collapse, shock, and death within hours). Hemoptysis, or coughing up blood, is a common symptom along with malaise and persistent fever. When the diagnosis is confirmed by x-ray, various laboratory studies such as blood counts, cultures of blood and sputum, and occasionally special blood tests for specific markers, are performed. Treatment with the appropriate antibiotics may com-mence, even before the specific causative germ is isolated. Frequently, treatment uses erythromycin-like drugs since they cover the majority of the most common pneumonia germs. Most cases of pneumonia are now treatable at home with ap-propriate antibiotics, rest, fluids, and symptomatic medicines for fever and cough. Follow-up is necessary to be sure the disease is cured.

Tuberculosis

Pulmonary tuberculosis is an infectious form of chronic pneumonia that used to be a major epidemic killer of the young and the poor, particularly in the teeming cities of the Industrial Revolution. It was spread from person to person by the airborne route. It is caused by a bacteria known as a Mycobacterium which survives well in sputum coughed up by victims and is the major mode of infection. After the discovery of streptomycin and other effective antibiotics, it was thought by the latter half of this century to be a disappearing disease, at least in the United States and other economically advantaged countries. An occasional case would pop up in an old person, whose childhood disease was reactivated by other illness, or an alcoholic or Third World immigrant. It was, until recently, easily and effectively treated. However, the proliferation of the homeless and the advent of AIDS has given new life to this old menace. Antibiotic-resistant strains of tuberculosis have emerged. Intense public health agency activity has resulted in some improvement in controlling the situation by detecting, isolating, and making sure of adequate treatment schedules for those who are infected. But, as of now, tuberculosis cannot be written off.

Diagnosis is made by chest x-ray and sputum examination and culture. The symptoms of tuberculosis are variable, but usually a chronic cough and malaise with associated fever and weight loss triggers the diagnostic evaluation. Some fungus pneumonias, such as valley fever (coccidioidomycosis) and histoplasmosis, caused by breathing in the fungus spores from contaminated dust, may have similar symptoms and must be differentiated from tuberculosis for appropriate antibiotic treatment.

Chronic Lung Disease, Emphysema, Chronic Obstructive Pulmonary Disease

Emphysema refers to the destruction of the alveoli with formation of larger "bubbles" of lung structure replacing the delicate alveolar sacules. The importance of this is simply that the gas-absorbing surface area is seriously decreased and oxygen–carbon dioxide exchange is decreased as a result. There are many causes of this disorder. The first is chronic inflammation, which breaks down the delicate alveolar wall. Second is infection, which does the same. A third is increased pressure required to exhale. These come about because of long-term abuse or insult to the respiratory tract. Finally, there are rare genetic types of emphysema.

Emphysema is an incapacitating and frequently fatal condition. It is, occasionally, unavoidable but is also, sadly, a frequent subsequence of our own doing. Smoking is our own choice, and air pollution is a result of the consumption of fuel for industry and transportation. The best bet is avoidance of the former and some type of control of the latter (easier said than done). Like obesity, the hope is with the young, if only they will heed the overwhelming evidence.

Management of chronic lung disease is best done by professionals but includes, in addition to avoidance of further damage from noxious inhalants, chronic oxygen therapy, judicious use of antibiotics and other medications, including bronchodilators and cortisone-type derivatives.

Asthma, the Wheezing Disease

The muscle of the tracheobronchial tree which underlies the mucus membrane is of the smooth or involuntary type. That is, it is not under our conscious control. The function of these muscle fibers is uncertain, but it is known that with inspiration, the muscle relaxes. With exhalation there is a certain amount of contraction normally; presumably to increase the pressure inside the alveoli to assist oxygen absorption. If bronchial muscle contraction is excessive, resistance to the airflow may cause exhalation difficulty and an audible noise, known as wheezing. This is the primary symptom of asthma. The bronchial muscular overcontraction is called bronchospasm. The bronchospasm is attributed to inflammation and oversensitivity of the bronchial membrane and smooth muscle to various negative stimuli including infection, allergens inhaled, ingested, or injected (pollens, dusts, bacteria, foods that one may be allergic to, insect stings, if one is allergic). This hypersensitive state may be inborn or acquired, but in any case may be mild and transient (outgrown) or late onset and progressive. Treatment, of course, depends upon the individual situation. Fortunately, we now have medications that may ameliorate and control bronchospasm. Unfortunately, because of ignorance or lack of adequate care, asthma as a disease has had worsening mortality statistics in recent years. This is shocking, since it seems to be avoidable most of the time.

The most useful treatments start with bronchodilators—medications that relax the bronchial muscles. These are administered via sprays, injection, or less effectively, ingestion. The sprays are best given via a "spacer" (e.g., Inspirease®), which breaks the spray into mist which more easily coats the membranes. The bronchodilators are actually adrenaline derivatives, which are powerful relaxers of smooth muscle. Many are available and are useful, but they are very potent and may have major side effects, particularly neuromuscular, with trembling and heart stimulation and palpitations. They are potentially hazardous if improperly used. The most important, and in the long term most effective, medications are the adrenocortical steroid preparations (steroids, cortisone derivatives). These adrenocortical hormone derivatives are powerful anti-inflammatory and anti-allergic agents. Although they do not immediately relax bronchospasm, as do the bronchodilators, they work to combat the cause of bronchospasm, the inflammation and oversensitivity of the bronchial tissues. If given on an emergency basis by injection, they may be life saving and may, within an hour or so, reverse a potentially fatal asthmatic attack. Of course, it is far better to prevent this; then radical measures are rarely required. It has become evident in recent years that the mainstay of treatment of chronic asthma is the judicious and persistent use of the inhaled steroid medication. Taken this way, even on a constant basis, few side effects or complications of chronic steroid use occur. The drug acts only on the bronchi and not enough is absorbed into the body to cause difficulties which could take place if the steroid preparations are taken regularly by mouth or injection. However, a short course of oral steroids may be necessary from time to time in serious flare-ups of chronic asthma. Other types of medications are occasionally used. These include theophylline, atropine, and expectorant formulations but the current consensus is that they are less effective than previously believed.

A word about expectorants: this term applies to those substances that liquefy, and make it easy to eliminate, the gummy, stringy, tough mucus, which can plug up the bronchial tubes and can literally choke us. This might be a problem with any disorder of the respiratory tree, but is especially important in asthma, pneumonia, bronchitis, and chronic pulmonary disease, such as chronic obstructive pulmonary disease and emphysema. The major liquifying remedy of the respiratory tract is plain water. Getting it to the mucus cells and into the mucus itself to thin it out is the problem. Drugs such as iodides, guaifenesin, and ammonium chloride have been used but their effectiveness is questionable. It appears that water is the key and the other substances are merely window dressing. Adequate hydration, and perhaps even mild overhydration, via tea, chicken soup, or whatever is the trick. My grandma's favorite was hot tea, lemon, 1 teaspoon of honey, and 1 tablespoon of brandy. My friend, the eminent pulmonologist and professor Irwin Ziment of UCLA, likes chili and other peppers. He opines that anything that stimulates the mucus glands, and peppers surely do, will increase flow, which is good. Most cough medications contain guaifenesin, which may or may not be helpful. High water intake is still of the greatest importance. Dehydration is a complication of respiratory and feverish illnesses of all kinds. Steam or vapor inhalation may feel good. Whether or not it does anything beneficial is also a matter of opinion.

Lung Cancer

It is bad news if you love your life, your wife, or your significant others. The great reservoir of smoking women seems to be the vanguard of an epidemic. Women seem to be more sensitive to airborne carcinogens. Also, although the smoking epidemic in the United States seems to have somewhat abated in adults, it smolders in our young population who are starting and continuing this lethal habit in increasing numbers. Smoking may not be the only cause of lung cancer, but it is by far the main culprit, and it is still unusual to see the disease in a nonsmoker. Other causes include noxious inhalants (asbestos, other silica particles, rock and coal dust in miners, radioactive gases such as radon). "Sidestream" or secondhand tobacco smoke also seems to be a factor, but this is still slightly controversial.

Lung cancer is best diagnosed early by chest x-ray. When it is detected this way, before symptoms develop, surgical removal is still curative much of the time. Statistics for such care have improved immensely in the past fifty years and chances of survival have increased from less than 10 percent to greater than 50 percent. Surgical techniques have become much more sophisticated, removing only part of the lung tissue instead of the entire lung being the usual procedure. Some types of lung cancer respond to chemotherapy and/or radiation therapy if surgery is not possible. Total cure without surgery is unlikely, but lengthy remissions do occur and, therefore, therapy is worth trying.

Since early diagnosis is the key, the question becomes, How often should routine chest x-rays be done? Such x-rays should definitely be taken when a persistent cough or upper respiratory infection doesn't clear up within a week or so. Also pneumonia, usually diagnosed by chest x-ray, must be checked by a repeat film three to four weeks later to make sure that the lung has cleared completely. Lung tumors often show up as a nonclearing opacity in the follow-up picture. Chest x-rays should be done at regular intervals (perhaps yearly) in people at risk, smokers, and individuals exposed to known hazardous materials. How often for the general population without specific indications? This question is controversial, particularly now in this age of medical cost containment. I believe that at least one baseline picture is advisable in the twenty-five to thirty-five-year-old group with periodic comparison films done every two to five years, depending upon age and other medical factors. A chest x-ray is quite useful for other baseline information (heart size and shape, bone structure) as well. Incidentally, bronchitis, asthma, and upper respiratory infections rarely produce abnormal x-ray findings. Emphysema and other chronic problems do, and our old (and reviving) nemesis, tuberculosis, requires an x-ray for proper diagnosis and treatment.

The CAT scan (computerized axial tomography) and MRI (magnetic resonance imaging) have revolutionized the diagnosis and management of lung and chest diseases of all kinds, including cancer. The doctor can determine the extent of the lesion, and also better plan the surgical approach. Bronchoscopy (looking into the tracheo-bronchial tree through a fiberoptic tube), done nowadays under anesthesia, is frequently of great help, and when combined with guided needle biopsy may confirm the diagnosis and reveal the type of tumor without subjecting the patient to open-chest surgery.

Smoking

I have alluded to the epidemic nature of this fatal addiction, noting the sad overabundance of new casualties of grade school and college age. On the other hand, there is good news. Perhaps there is no more remarkable epidemiological success story than that of the battle to create a "Smoke-Free America." During my youth, tobacco smoking was associated with manliness, maturity, success in sports, and all good things of life! Our greatest heroes and role models—President Franklin

Roosevelt, Humphrey Bogart, Gary Cooper—all were chain-smokers. We smoked as soon as we could get away with it. We smoked in college classrooms, even in medical school. Medical conventions were full of tobacco company booths giving doctors free samples. What a change in the last few decades! The great majority of American adults consider smokers pariahs. That the idea has gotten across is in itself an amazing development.

By now, the hazards of smoking have been driven into our consciousness from all sides, so I will not further belabor this issue. Rather, I will relate my own experience. I stopped my own habit of three packs per day, seven years ago. I was addicted as anyone might be after forty years. As a physician, I had special pressures to quit aimed my way. My major motivation to stop, however, was ego driven. I resented my own stubbornness and inability to control this self-destructive appetite which was so detrimental to my social, professional, and physical health. I had enjoyed, despite smoking, excellent health (or so I thought), never having missed a day of work (macho stupidity, in retrospect). A severe case of bronchitis was the turning point. Nothing, not food, nor drink, nor smoking, tasted good. I took advantage of this disinclination by stopping cold turkey. The subsequent withdrawal discomfort was indistinguishable from the misery of the upper respiratory infection. When I recovered from that, I discovered a brighter new existence. Not only did the nagging from my wife, my patients, my family, and my colleagues cease, but my nose cleared for the first time in forty years. I had thought I had hay fever! The tendency to cough violently from minor irritations went away. I saved much money (cigarette prices have skyrocketed; my habit cost $6.00 per day back then) and spent it on gratifying things, such as smoke-free travel and restaurants (no hassling), unburned new clothes, and very appreciative friends who no longer either had to avoid or abide me. To be sure, I occasionally miss, even dream of, my old smoky companion, but not enough to resume what was in retrospect a miserable slavery. Since my experience, I have accentuated the strong positive features of quitting to my smoking friends and patients, rather than recounting the usual horror stories. Even so, we converts are not yet out of the woods. The incidence of lung cancer and other serious pulmonary and cardiovascular disease is higher in us than in those who never smoked, but the statistics improve the further we get from the time of cessation. Best of all, I'm proud of myself—I kicked the habit.

I suppose I should be proud because it is estimated that only 2 to 3 percent of addicted smokers are able to quit each year, despite the aid of sedatives, antidepressants, nicotine patches, and nicotine gum. The major requirement for success is determination to quit in spite of the threat of discomfort and weight gain. (It's far healthier to gain weight than to continue to smoke.) So, sadly, we continue to reap the deadly harvest—some 400,000 tobacco-related deaths in 1995 (one of them my own sister).

DR. DASHE'S TIPS FOR HEALTH MAINTENANCE

1. Quit smoking. I know, easier said than done, but it kills more people in one year in the United States than were killed in the four years of the Civil War.

2. Reduce your exposure to airborne pollutants. If you live in a metropolitan area keep advised of air quality conditions and exercise appropriate precautions.

3. The common cold will be your most frequent contact with respiratory infection. Ranging from annoying to miserable it is a fact of life and will be cured by time and soothed by easily-acquired medications.

4. More serious infections of the bronchi (bronchitis) and lungs (pneumonia) have specific causes and treatments with various antibiotics. The pneumonia vaccines are available and strongly recommended.

5. True influenza is a serious respiratory infection that is preventable by vaccination and treatable with antiviral drugs.

6. Asthma afflicts almost 13 million Americans; if you have it you can still live an active and healthy life. The rising death toll due to asthma is completely avoidable if people just play an active role in their health care maintenance.

7. Sleep apnea syndrome, due to upper respiratory obstruction, may be manifested not only by loud snoring but more importantly interrupted sleep and daytime grogginess and fatigue. In the worst cases, the nocturnal oxygen deprivation may cause serious heart problems. Detection and treatment, usually with continuous positive air pressure (C-PAP) and less commonly with surgery, are very effective.

8. However, snoring is mostly a tremendous bother, especially for your partner, but mostly harmless unless connected with sleep apnea.

9. If you smoke you would be wise to get regular chest x-rays for lung cancer detection. Your survival will depend on early detection.

10. Chronic lung disease (including emphysema) is the end result of years of damage to the lungs. Once developed, it is incapacitating but treatable. It is far better to avoid it by stopping smoking.

Chapter 8

SKIN AND HAIR

What is the largest grouping of human tissues into a distinct structure that performs distinct tasks and is a major instrument of multiple vital actions? If you guessed the skin is the largest organ of the body, you would have been right. The skin organ has many functions other than covering your insides.

Functions of the Skin

Heating and Cooling Mechanism

The skin is richly supplied with a capillary network capable of expanding and contracting the blood flow underneath. This is of major importance, since our internal body temperature cannot vary more than a few degrees for very long without harm to our tissues (normal range is from 98 degrees to 100 degrees F). When hot, we "flush" and sweat. Blood has been automatically shunted toward the surface, where cooling may take place, because the arterioles expand. This heat exchange is abetted by the evaporation of our sweat, somewhat like a "swamp cooler." The capillaries and sweat glands, which are really little salt and water pumps, respond via automatic (autonomic) signals from the central nervous system and, upon command, pour liquid onto our surfaces.

The opposite happens when we are too cool. The autonomic nervous system shunts the blood from the skin, by contracting the arterioles, to the center of the body and the brain, heart, and kidneys. Hence the pallor and even bluish tinge of our surfaces when we are cold. Sweating also ceases. Of course, when the cold deprives the skin of nourishing blood for too long, the serious condition known as frostbite may occur.

Lubricating Mechanism

The skin is supplied in most areas not only by sweat glands but also oil glands, which secrete a lubricating substance known as sebum (hence the name sebaceous glands). This material lubricates the skin and keeps it and the tissue beneath from drying out. The process is known as exocrine or apocrine secretion, as opposed to endocrine, wherein the glands deliver their products, called hormones, directly into the bloodstream. Sebum varies in thickness from very light oil to heavy wax, as in the ear canals, depending upon the needs of the area lubricated. Without this lubricant, our skin would dry and crack and vital fluids would be lost from the body.

Another apocrine function is rather intriguing. That is odor production. It has long been recognized that in lower life forms, both plant and animal, odors may be produced that serve as a repellent (angry skunk) or attractant (musk scents). Some odors, called pheromones, are known sexual attractants secreted by either or both sexes. These potent fragrances may be so subtle that they may not even be recognizable as an odor, but they are of major importance in mate selection in many species (apparently including humans). Fresh apocrine secretion in humans is practically odorless unless flavored by something we eat, such as garlic. It, however, contains substances that either attract or repel potential sexual partners. Pheromones also stimulate endocrine function. The primitive part of the brain known as the olfactory system or "smell brain" detects the pheromone. This signals, via the central nervous system wiring, the neuroendocrine part of the brain known as the hypothalamus. It is capable of secreting a hormone known as GNRF (gonadotrophin releasing factor). This hormone signals the adjacent pituitary gland to secrete sex-gland-stimulating hormones, which finally signal the testes in the man and the ovaries in the woman, to get busy and "do their thing." The reverse process also occurs; that is, sex hormones stimulate pheromone production.

The eccrine (exocrine) system, particularly the sebaceous glands (also known as apocrine glands), is also under the influence not only of the central nervous system but also the endocrine glands. For instance, increased thyroid hormone production by the thyroid gland will stimulate sweating, a frequent symptom of overactivity. The sebaceous glands are stimulated by the sex hormones, particularly male hormones (androgens), either testosterone from the sex glands or androsterones from the adrenal glands. This is why oily skin and acne do not occur before puberty and decrease in older ages as the hormone production falls.

Truly foul odors are not produced by normal skin; they require bacterial action on unwashed skin, which takes time. The best preventive is soap and water. Deodorants, which occasionally also prevent sweating, are mere stopgaps. However, some folks enjoy day-old, even riper aromas. To each his or her own. Napoleon was said to have written to Josephine from the front, "Don't wash. I'm coming home next week!"

Disorders and Management of the Skin and Hair

Apocrine Glands

Problems may occur with the apocrine glands. Both sweat and sebaceous glands have ducts (tubes) leading to the surface from the location beneath (about ⅛ to ½ inch). The apocrine glands frequently empty into a hair follicle. If the sweat gland duct is blocked, it produces what is generally called a whitehead; if it is a sebaceous blockage it produces a blackhead (comedone). Bacterial invasion of a blocked apocrine gland will lead to acne of a greater or lesser degree. A staphylococcus germ may cause a severe infection known familiarly as a boil or medically as a furuncle or skin abscess. A chronic smoldering, less acute infection may produce a red, bumpy eruption known as acne rosacea. If it affects the skin of the nose it causes an embarrassing, clownlike, W. C. Fields proboscis known as rhinophyma; this is very disfiguring and is *not* related to alcohol. A very slow and chronic infection of the glands causes a red, flaky rash known as seborrhea. In the scalp, seborrhea is the cause of dandruff. Acne (the medical term is acne vulgaris) is a very common skin condition affecting just about all adolescents. The bumps, blackheads, and little boils most frequently involve the face, neck, and chest. The basic problem again involves increased production of androgen-generated sebum with blockage of the opening of the glands causing the characteristic zit. The action of skin bacteria on the sebum leads to inflammation and scarring (both physical and psychological). Although generally self-limited, beginning at puberty and ending at adulthood, acne occasionally persists well into maturity.

Management of these apocrine disorders depends, of course, upon the type and particular manifestation. Most of these problems, if unresponsive to common home remedies, require medical consultation. In any case, keep your hands off, and avoid picking, squeezing, and scratching, which usually only makes things worse. Abscesses may require surgical drainage if they don't open spontaneously or after warm, wet compresses are applied, but simple acne may respond to good hygiene (faithful scrubbing with plenty of soap and water, especially germicidal soaps such as Phisohex and the like) and various drying agents available over the counter. Seborrhea may require prescription medicines but various milder dandruff shampoos (Selsun Blue®, Head & Shoulders) usually are sufficient. Regular daily use of germicidal soaps (Phisohex) in particularly susceptible spots, especially the groin, between the buttocks, armpits, face, and back may prevent recurrent boils. Showering once or twice a day works wonders! Severe acne responds well to more powerful medically prescribed treatments, including internal or external antibiotic application. In my experience, Cleocin® lotion application is very effective. Strong external skin peeling agents such as vitamin A derivatives (Accutane® taken orally or Retin-A® applied to the skin surface) are powerful remedies. Seborrhea, likewise, may respond to these very potent agents, which must be medically monitored.

Hyperhidrosis

Excessive sweating, or hyperhidrosis, is a vexing and embarrassing symptom suffered by some individuals, men more often than women. The cause is usually unknown, although it may be due to another underlying disease such as hyperthyroidism (overactive thyroid) or severe chronic anxiety. If an underlying cause is present, treatment of the primary disorder will cure the sweating problem as well. If it is not, it becomes a frustrating matter with which to deal. There are potent antisweating chemicals that may be applied to severely affected areas such as armpits and palms. These are aluminum chloride preparations (Drysol®, Xerac®). Occasionally, judicious use of mild tranquilizers may help, but other medicines such as dry-up pills (atropine drugs) aren't very useful in most cases. I have had patients who have claimed that this symptom has ruined their lives; they cannot even bear to shake hands for fear of offending by offering a wet, limp paw. These drastic situations occasionally call for drastic measures, including the severing of the autonomic nerves to the extremities (sympathectomy). In addition, there are several other means of dealing with this problem. Biofeedback, an alternative medical practice, has been claimed to be effective in some cases. (I personally have not seen any great success, but I have heard some favorable anecdotes; no harm done in any case.) Another procedure, known as iontopheresis, or the application of an electric current to the sweat glands, has been advocated. Again, I have no personal experience, but it is another harmless remedy offered by some dermatologists.

Bromhidrosis

Foul body odor, or bromhidrosis, is another serious social problem for some victims. It is actually rare other than when caused by poor hygiene. Normal apocrine sweat is odorless unless certain foods (for example, garlic) are eaten and partially excreted by the skin. Sweat and sebum will smell fetid if acted upon by normal body bacteria after a day or so. Really bad odor requires time to evolve. Very rarely true bromhidrosis, despite showering, will occur in some genetically cursed persons. There are measures that may ameliorate this, and medical consultation is in order.

Psoriasis

This is a mysterious and frustrating disorder of unknown cause. It is common, afflicting about four million Americans and about 2 percent of the world's population. More men than women are affected and there is a definite hereditary disposition. This is a chronic disease, and is rarely transient, although often it disappears only to reappear for no apparent reason; perhaps stress or anxiety may be precipitating factors. The rash of psoriasis consists, usually, of slightly raised, red, flaky, scaly plaques which may occur anywhere on the body. The elbows, knees, and face are most commonly affected. It rarely affects the whole body nor is it very severe or incapacitating. Occasionally, along with the rash, systemic symptoms, such as arthritis, especially in the hands, feet, neck, and lower back, may occur. Sometimes blood abnormalities, such as high cholesterol and high uric acid, may be present. The rash usually is seen as sharply demarcated areas of almost any size. Itching occurs only in about 20 percent of victims. Scaling may not be apparent until the surface is scratched, when the silvery flakes appear. Fingernails may appear pitted and discolored. Psoriasis may be very embarrassing.

I cannot emphasize too strongly that psoriasis is a treatable disease and optimism is warranted. Treatment does require some patience and encouragement, for it is occasionally awkward and slightly messy. This includes application of steroid creams or other topical applications, including injection by the doctor of steroids under the skin. Decolorized coal tar applications are very effective, particularly when used with midrange ultraviolet light application (UVB). Repeated exposure to sunlight or the middle-wave-length UVB may clear up many cases. More aggressive treatment is rarely necessary, but is available and effective if a dermatologist carries it out. Severe psoriasis and psoriatic arthritis requires intense specialized care and treatment includes effective medications which are potentially dangerous and need careful monitoring by an expert.

Baldness

I told you that this is a book about male medical maladies, so here's a dilly: hair loss. Not that it is actually limited to us, since females, too, are occasionally sufferers of this humiliating disorder, but wigs do look nicer on them. I am told by psychologists and sex therapists that hair loss is the major presenting concern of the male patient seeking help and guidance.

Male pattern baldness is an outcome of the action of male hormones on the hair follicle, a genetic predetermination with a variable penetrance, or timetable. Genetic traits are present at conception, but the timing of the expression of the trait is determined by other factors, such as time of life, nutrition, stress levels, and so on. This is the meaning of the term *penetrance*. Male pattern baldness generally starts in the twenties and thirties and affects the frontal areas first, creating the familiar "Nixon horns." Hair loss on top begins, less noticeably, at about the same time with the cowlick area. Depending upon the genetic predisposition, the process will continue more or less until, in the worst-case scenario, the frontal and central bald portions join, leaving a fringe along the sides and back. Some cultures, notably Japanese, consider this very sexy and some Japanese men, in times past, shaved their heads in this pattern to provide a more fierce, warrior look. Alas, this is not the case in usual Western circles, although various styles and degrees of baldness, self-induced, are sometimes considered fashionable (such as with the late Yul Brynner and Telly Savalas). Baldness does not occur with any frequency in certain groups (for example, Native Americans) or in castrated or eunuchoid men. The genetic pattern is not entirely certain either; one is not always fated to have the hairline of one's father, but the final result is dependent upon one's heritage one way or another. I have often wondered if Mother Nature is mocking me and my brothers by taking the hair from our heads and sticking it in our noses and ears. It ain't funny, Mother!

Short of castration, there is little that can be done by medical science to prevent male pattern baldness. Basic good hair care is important to avoid aggravating the condition. This includes keeping the hair and scalp clean without using harsh shampoos or too-frequent shampooing; avoidance of physical abuse to hair follicles such as some straightening techniques and solutions; and avoidance of hairstyles that pull on the hair, which may permanently damage the follicles. Conditioning rinses may help damaged hair. Despite the many claims for hair restorers, there are few that have been scientifically tested and found to be effective, except for minoxidil (Rogaine®) and finasteride (Propecia® and Proscar®, identical drugs with different names) (see under Prostate, page 187).

Rogaine, now available without prescription, is a curious antihypertensive medication that was found by accident to cause, as an unwanted side effect, abnormal hair growth all over. This serendipitous finding led to the development of a topical lotion which, when applied daily and regularly, seems to retard loss and even, occasionally, restore hair growth in men and women. It works to some degree in about 40 to 50 percent of cases and is worth trying. It is, unfortunately, rather expensive. It has been released over the counter and seems to be quite safe, if used as directed. Propecia (actually half-strength Proscar) blocks the conversion of testosterone to dihydrotestosterone, thereby blocking the tendency to male baldness (see under Prostate, page 187). Unfortunately it may be a mild sexual downer by virtue of this hormonal action.

The only other truly restorative maneuvers are surgical; that is, plastic surgery. Hair plug grafts, which are small plugs of scalp, are removed from hairy areas on the sides and back of the head and implanted directly into the bald areas in front and on top. They work, although at first the rows of plugs give the appearance of a Kansas cornfield in early spring. Eventually they grow out to give a slightly thin but acceptable crop. Other plastic surgical procedures, such as replacing lateral scalp hair toward the top by stagewise excision of the bald spot, may provide some cosmetic relief. These plastic surgeries, by the way, are rather expensive indeed, so if you're poor, consider a Michael Jordan "do."

Various other cosmetic buys (hair pieces, weaving, and so on) tend to be pretty good (and expensive) or bad (grotesque). Many women, incidentally, think bald men are sexier than the hirsute; and why not; they have proven that they have an abundance of testosterone.

There are other types of hair loss, which are far less common and are true disease states, unlike garden-variety baldness. Alopecia, which means hair loss, may occur with a variety of systemic or skin diseases. For instance, a severe infection may cause temporary, or in extreme cases permanent, total hair loss. Drugs, notably those used in chemotherapy, may do the same, although this type of general alopecia is almost always temporary. Local infection, such as ringworm, a fungus of the scalp, will cause patchy alopecia which is reversible with treatment. A mysterious condition known as alopecia areata, which is also a patchy type of hair loss (on the head) is probably a form of allergy and may respond to anti-allergy treatments such as steroid applications. Finally, there are sporadic and peculiar episodes of hair loss, usually of the head hair and sometimes the whole body (alopecia totalis), that defy explanation and may be permanent. Some experts believe that stress and psychologic factors, such as shock, may be responsible, but this explanation is still controversial and in any case, there is no treatment.

Warts

These are hard and ragged little bumps which are actually benign skin tumors that are caused by viruses known as human papilloma viruses. They are rarely anything more than a bother and a fright to men (who always think of cancer) although they can be disfiguring and mildly incapacitating, especially if they involve the extremities, face, or genitals (genital warts are a different matter and are dealt with in the chapter on sexually transmitted disease). Warts have a long folk history and remedies have varied from swinging a dead cat around by the tail ten times in the village square at midnight (Mark Twain) to application of the fat of a lion (Galen). Actually, many things do work, including electric needle desiccation or liquid nitrogen application. Almost everything works, I found. See the doctor—forget the cat.

Athlete's Foot and Groin (Jock Itch)

Fungi are indeed among us and these primitive plant forms just love our dark, moist, rubbing spaces (between the toes and in the groin). These annoying rashes are easily treated with the many effective fungicidal creams available (Lotrimin, Naftate®). One can prevent them by keeping these moist dark areas dry, clean, and powdered, particularly in hot weather. It is useless to worry about catching a fungus in the gym; they are here, there, and everywhere, just waiting for a playground.

Skin Cancer

Frying your largest organ with dangerous electromagnetic waves is probably the last thing you would want to do, if you think of it this way. Yet we inflict this horror upon ourselves, usually out of narcissistic naiveté, but more frequently stubborn denial. I refer to the quaint custom known as tanning. We even pay for it; hence, the growing incidence of skin malignancy in our population. The skin malignancy known as melanoma has become a plague of near epidemic proportions. The gloomy projection of the dermatologic epidemiologist is that the incidence is growing at a rapid rate; presumably partly because of the loss of much of our protective atmospheric ozone layer. Experts estimate now that skin cancers will affect one out of every seven people, with increasing frequency in the future. I cringe whenever I pass a beach where I see my poor fellow humans, unfortunately mostly youngsters, turning themselves over and over as if they are lambs on a spit.

In case I have not made the point clear enough, let me suggest to the young, bronzed Adonis that protection is what your largest organ really needs. If you cannot abide the shade, use a potent sunscreen, at least SPF 15. Melanoma is a particularly deadly cancer; it spreads rapidly via the bloodstream and thus far little effective treatment is available if it is not caught before it spreads. It is truly a terrible thing to see people in their thirties and forties succumb. The other skin cancers related to solar ultraviolet exposures, namely basal cells and squamous cells, are less malignant but frequently are quite disfiguring and, at times, difficult to treat.

The best way to deal with skin cancer is to prevent it and not have to deal with it at all, but short of this, early detection is of great importance. Fortunately, skin cancers are superficial to begin with and usually can be easily seen. Periodic inspection of your visible surfaces is a good idea; microscopic inspection is not necessary (Figure 8-1). Hidden areas such as your back are best inspected by your loved one. The places where "the sun don't shine" are thankfully spared from solar mischief, but even there skin tumors may appear.

Moral: Check with your doctor if lumps or bumps or color changes are noted. Better be safe—check it out with the doctor.

Wrinkles and Age Spots

As we age, our skin changes (as if you hadn't noticed). Our skin is at its best during infancy when it is soft yet firm, pliable, unblemished, and of even color; like a baby's bottom as it were. It's downhill from there for various reasons. Aging itself provides most of the change. The liquid content of the skin gradually de-

---

Figure 8-1: SKIN DANGER SIGNS

Look for danger signs in pigmented lesions of the skin. Consult your dermatologist immediately if any of your moles or pigmented spots exhibit:

A   **Asymmetry**—one half unlike the other half.

B   **Border irregular**—scalloped or poorly circumscribed border.

C   **Color varied**—from one area to another; shades of tan and brown; black; sometimes white, red, or blue.

D   **Diameter larger**—than 6 millimeters as a rule (the diameter of a pencil eraser)

Mind these ABCDs. They may be signs of malignant melanoma.

---

creases and the tissues lose firmness as desiccation and gravity take their toll. The radiation of the sun, as does all radiation, has cumulative effects. That is, it all adds up; you don't get to go back to square one after you lose that sunburn. The net effect of this is what we all discover with horror someday when we look in the mirror. I prefer to call my changes freckles, character lines, and character sculpturing. Unless you are a clone of Oscar Wilde's *Dorian Gray*, whose portrait aged while he remained as youthful as Michael Jackson, you are going to face this sometime or other. But is there something to be done? Of course there is. We have wrinkle creams and plastic surgery. Before we go into these, please recall that the sun is largely responsible for pigmentary blemishes and leathering of our exposed areas, so prevention by protective measures is of paramount importance.

Once the spots and wrinkles have formed, there are some apparently effective peeling agents that may work by removing superficial layers of skin and replacing them with younger-appearing, deeper layers. These substances vary in strength and effectiveness but they all work by acting as dermal irritants. The medications used range from the weaker nonprescription alpha-hydroxy acid preparations (Alpha Hydrox®) to the prescription strength tretinoin (Renova®). Even stronger are more abrasive agents such as laser beams, chemical exfoliants such as flurouracil, and dermabrasion, which actually uses sanding wheels. None of this is miraculous, to be sure, but in the patients I have seen, some improvement in pigmentation and fine wrinkling is apparent. For deep wrinkles and sags, one must call upon plastic surgeons. Women have, historically, availed themselves of cosmetic surgery far more often than men. This is no longer the case; many men wish to have their appearance improved by skin tightening, jowl erasing, flab deflating by liposuction, or deep wrinkles ironing. So go ahead, if this is important enough to warrant the expense and discomfort of such surgery, which is, by and large, reasonably safe if done by a reliable, certified plastic surgeon. Ask your trusted physician for a referral.

General Care of the Skin

If you haven't already surmised, skin care is based upon common sense and the principles of moderation. Cleanliness is most important. Good nutrition and sensible practices of hygiene in daily living supersede any advertising claim for skin products. Avoidance of harmful chemicals and excessive sunlight is all that is necessary to keep your largest organ happy and healthy. Too much of a good thing is also unwise; too frequent washing may lead to removal of protective natural oils and lubricants and may require lubricating emollients for relief. Everyone is different and no specific regimen applies to all.

Finally, a word about the specialty of dermatology. I have been struck by the richness and splendor of dermatologic disease nomenclature. In the past, every little rash had a marvelous Latin name of its own. Examples include pityriasis rosea, nevus flammeus, melasma, lentigines, granuloma annulare, erythema multiforme, etc. My moribund dermatologist friend whispered to me toward the end, "I didn't know what caused the damn things, so I gave them great names." And so it goes, still, with much of medicine. But we try, and slowly we are getting to know what these things mean, and then we can give them simpler names.

DR. DASHE'S TIPS FOR HEALTH MAINTENANCE

1. Skin care has long been associated with women, but men are now becoming more interested in taking care of their skin. Makes sense, it's the largest organ of the body and performs vital functions including environmental protection and temperature regulation.

2. The skin is full of glands that keep us cool and protected. Acute infections (boils or abscesses) and chronic ones (seborrhea or rosacea) are common problems, and a dermatologist is well equipped to provide some or total relief from these maladies.

3. Acne is the bane of youth and a byproduct of raging sex hormones; proper cleansing can help decrease the incidence and protect skin from infections.

4. Chronic skin eruptions, including the most common, psoriasis, can be successfully treated with cortisone and other potent medications.

5. Athlete's foot is another common fungus that affects mostly men. Keep your feet dry and expose them to air when you get done with your day or your activity. Fungus loves a damp dark place to live and you're doing it a favor by keeping your sweaty socks on all day. There are some effective over-the-counter medicines as well as more potent prescription medications available.

6. Skin cancer is an increasingly frequent problem, and the incidence of deadly melanoma is frightening. If you are out in the sun, especially if you are fair in complexion, cover up with clothes or sunblock.

7. Self examination is a good way to spot possible skin cancer; early detection is important to ensure that it doesn't get worse and that scarring is minimized.

8. Baldness is preventable by castration. Not a viable alternative for most, so we are left only with minoxidil, finasteride, plastic surgery, or a toupee to deal with our shiny pates.

9. Wrinkles and age spots are the unavoidable results of time and can be dealt with using various methods from chemical to surgical. More and more men are finding that they are happy with the results of brow lifts and face tucks.

10. A healthy lifestyle can do the most to ensure that your skin remains trouble free and properly functioning.

Chapter 9

THE ENDOCRINE SYSTEM

Ah, for the good old days of delivering babies, sewing up wounds, and treating malaria, fractures, and common colds as Medical Officer of the Day in the Air Force.

This is my way of telling you that, despite my lifelong admiration for the marvelous functional design and workings of the human body, still, as my career progressed I realized that one cannot be an expert in everything. I owed it to my patients to have more knowledge about less rather than less about more. My particular choice of specialization evolved finally into the field of endocrinology: the study of the glands of internal secretion and the diseases stemming from their deficiency or malfunction, an important branch of internal medicine, and my major field.

The two systems that regulate all of our elegant and complex body functioning are the central nervous system and the endocrine system. Up until a half century ago, they were thought to be separate systems. We know now that they are closely interrelated and the field of neuroendocrinology has become one of great interest and importance. For the sake of this short book, however, we will separate the two and discuss the major endocrine glands, their duties, and their disorders.

The "Masters"

The pituitary gland sits at the base of the brain. If you took a pencil (don't try this at home) and stuck it about 4 inches up into your nose, you would run smack into it. About sixty years ago, it was given the title of "master gland." It produced the chemicals we call hormones which, when released into the bloodstream by the gland, seemed to control the other glands, including the thyroid gland (in the neck), the adrenal glands (on top of the kidneys), and the sex glands (testes in the male, ovaries in the female). Gradually, other pituitary hormones were discovered. Growth hormone is one which stimulates the growth of our bones and soft tissues and thereby our height. The hormone prolactin is necessary for production of milk in the new mother. A hormone from the posterior (back part) of the pituitary, vasopressin, gives the kidneys the ability to concentrate urine, so that we do not lose too much body fluid and become dehydrated. This actually liberates us air-breathing creatures from the sea, from where all land animals originated. Sea animals do not require vasopressin. They do not dehydrate in their liquid world.

In the past fifty years or so it has been found that the pituitary gland is not an "independent contractor." Indeed, it has its own master. A part of the brain known as the hypothalamus controls much of the pituitary functioning with its own set of hormone signalers. The hypothalamus, in turn, has attachments to the rest of the brain, which may regulate the hypothalamic action. This explains why emotional stresses can affect our hormonal functions. For example, emotional stress may cause our adrenal glands to put out stress hormones, such as adrenaline and cortisone. The sight of a lovely woman may cause an acute rise in the male's testosterone levels. These rather dramatic events are simple illustrations of only a few of the constant and multiple functions of our neuroendocrine system.

The Peripheral Glandular System

Thyroid

The thyroid gland, which lies in the neck just in front of the trachea (Figure 9-1), is a 1-to-2-ounce structure which is under the control of the pituitary gland. The pituitary gland makes thyroid stimulating hormone (TSH). TSH stimulates the thyroid gland to make and release thyroid hormone (called thyroxin) into the bloodstream. Thyroxin's major function is to regulate our general metabolism, including heat production, energy burning, muscular activity, brain action, and so on. Without adequate thyroid hormone we become hypothyroid (hypo = down, hyper = up). Symptoms of hypothyroidism include fatigue, weakness, lethargy, feeling cold, and mental sluggishness. With thyroid overactivity or hyperthyroidism, the reverse is the case, with overactivity, jumpy muscles, higher temperature (and feeling hot), and irritability. Taking excessive thyroid hormone by mouth, which people occasionally do, can be dangerous. This is an unfortunate error by patient or doctor or both; this hormone was and is being used erroneously and indiscriminately for nonthyroid conditions such as overweight and chronic fatigue.

Tumors and nodules of the thyroid gland are, fortunately, relatively easy to detect, since they generally are visible or palpable due to their prominent location. Diseases of the thyroid in general are not hard to treat if properly diagnosed and the doctor either knows how or gets help from a qualified endocrine specialist.

Common Diseases of the Thyroid Gland

Goiter—simple or nodular. Goiter means thyroid gland enlargement, which may have many different causes. For many years, doctors thought that this condition occurs as a consequence of iodine deficiency in the diet. The element iodine is necessary for the production of thyroid hormone; it is a major component. There is plenty of iodine in foods available in areas close to the ocean but people living in landlocked, inland regions may have iodine-deficient diets and goiters may result. There are famous old *National Geographic* photos of tribes with huge swollen

Figure 9-1: THE ENDOCRINE SYSTEM

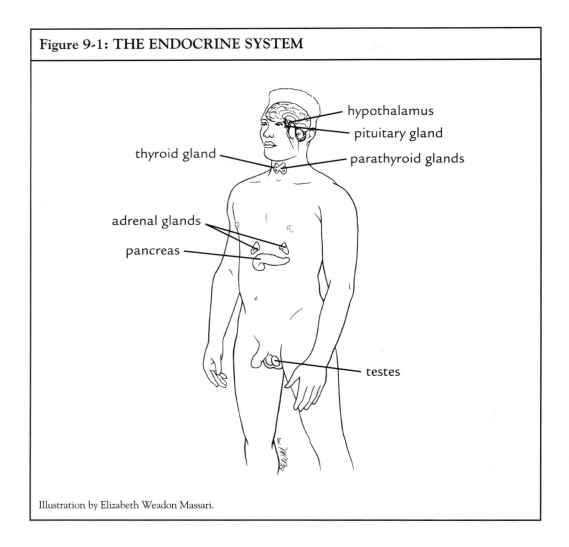

Illustration by Elizabeth Weadon Massari.

necks. It is for this reason that common table salt was, and still is, iodized. It became obvious, however, over the past forty to fifty years, that iodine deficiency was not responsible for most cases of goiter seen in the Western world. As a matter of fact, some cases of goiter are caused or aggravated by iodine, and in general iodized salt and other foods containing large amounts of it (kelp or seaweed, shellfish) should be avoided by people with goiters or a strong family history of them. Most goiters are familial, as is much thyroid disease. Oddly enough, the genetic propensity to thyroid disease is not uniform; that is, any and all assorted thyroid problems tend to run in the same family tree. We don't know why this is, but experts think that many thyroid disorders begin with inherited enzyme deficiencies in the manufacture of thyroid hormone. This seems to trigger the disease process. Giving thyroid hormone is the treatment; it works much of the time.

Autoimmune inflammatory disease of the thyroid gland. Allergy to one's own thyroid tissue may result from congenital disease, producing thyroiditis of various types. These include Hashimoto's thyroiditis with irregular goiter and Graves' disease (the most common cause of hyperthyroidism or overactivity of the thyroid gland). Antithyroid antibodies are often found in these diseases. Treatment depends upon the precise diagnosis. For Graves' disease, for instance, which is manifested by symptoms of overactivity, treatment is usually instituted with antithyroid medication such as PTU (propylthiouracil) or methimazole (Tapizole®). Frequently, oral administration of radioactive iodine treatment is used to quiet the overactivity by internal radiation—a more permanent form of treatment that is favored by some endocrinologists. Hashimoto's thyroiditis, which is closely related to Graves' disease, usually does not cause overactivity but it frequently does cause a goiter and occasionally hypothyroidism. This disorder is nicely treated with administration of thyroid hormone, levothyroxine (Synthroid®, Levothyroid®, and others), which suppresses the process and the goiter and replaces the deficiency of thyroid hormone, if it exists. Incidentally, generic hormone preparations, including thyroid hormone, should be avoided. Biostandardization is occasionally poor and accurate dosing may be impossible.

Thyroid nodules—single or multiple. These are worrisome—what worries us, of course, is the question of malignancy. Let me say right off that multiple nodular changes of the thyroid are usually not cancerous, so a multiple nodular goiter is better to present to your doctor than a simple nodule. A solitary nodule requires immediate attention, particularly if there is any history of radiation exposure during the early years of life. The children exposed to the Chernoble disaster, for instance, have a terribly high incidence of nodules and cancer of the thyroid because of the immense amount of radioactive iodine released during that tragic event. American children of years past were exposed to x-ray therapy of the head and neck for treatment of such things as acne or tonsil enlargement, and in the thirties, forties, and fifties, every shoe store had a foot fluoroscope machine where your child could stand and have x-rays of the feet to check toe room (and at the same time, get testicles, head, and neck nicely irradiated!). The machines were outlawed in the fifties. Solitary thyroid nodules may be solid or fluid-filled cysts. The diagnosis has been simplified and made far more accurate by the use of the rapid, painless fine-needle biopsy. It is done in about thirty seconds as an office procedure. If a fluid-filled cyst is present, physical and emotional relief is instantaneous. These cysts are almost always benign and when drained through the needle, they disappear. (They can recur and require repeat drainage.) If the nodule is solid, tissue juice and a few cells are removed, usually enough for the pathologist to examine microscopically and determine whether it is benign (as it is most of the time) or not. Sometimes the results are equivocal but if so, surgery is usually recommended. Occasionally, a period of a few months of observation and treatment with thyroxine is tried, to see if the nodule will shrink or go away. Close follow-up and observation is necessary, obviously. Treatment for malignant thyroid nodules consists of total removal of the gland followed, usually, by a cancer-ablating dose of radioiodine to kill all remaining thyroid cells, cancerous or not. Lifelong supplementation with thyroid hormone then commences, and in greater than 90 percent of cases, the patient is cured. As cancers go, this tends to be a nice one. It has been said that the major cause of death in thyroid cancer victims is automobile accidents; that is, they don't die from their thyroid cancer but rather from something else.

Adrenals

The adrenal glands are small, triangular objects that lie on top of the kidneys. These little structures are actually two glands in one, with the central core (medulla) manufacturing and releasing on command adrenaline (or epinephrines, to be more precise). Epinephrines (there are actually several types) are the immediate fight-or-flight-inducing hormones. They are the culprits that raise your blood pressure, get your blood sugar (and your courage) up, elevate your heart rate, curl your lip, widen your nostrils, raise your hackles and, if you are smart, enable you to get the hell out of the situation!

The outer shell (cortex) of the adrenal gland is totally different and is under the control of the pituitary gland via that structure's hormone, ACTH (adrenocortical-trophic hormone). ACTH acts upon the adrenal cortex to produce three different hormones: 1) cortisone (actually hydrocortisone) which has a stress reaction function, including keeping our blood sugar and pressure up and preventing needless inflammation; 2) mineral-regulating hormones (this function keeps our blood salts in balance); and 3) androgen (male hormone). Adrenal androgens are peculiar; they are produced in both sexes. They are not as potent as testosterone but they are responsible for growth of the hair in the armpits, pubis, and so on (especially in women). The importance of this is uncertain, but too much of this hormone can be trouble in the woman (but not in men who are hirsute anyway).

Tumors and overactivity of the adrenal glands are relatively rare conditions and require complex and sophisticated tests and treatments. Masculinization (virilization), excessive hair, increased muscle, genital enlargement, and increased libido, will scarcely be noticed or minded by us men, but when it occurs in a woman or a child, it is a real disaster. This almost always is due to adrenal cortex overproduction of androgen and requires proper diagnosis and treatment. Overproduction of cortisone, on the contrary, produces a serious condition known as Cushing's syndrome. Dr. Harvey Cushing was among the first to describe this syndrome, which is manifested by severe muscle weakness and wasting, central obesity, and "buffalo hump" (a fatty bulging of the upper back). Many of the circus sideshow freaks, such as the bearded lady and some dwarfs, are products of endocrine disease.

Parathyroids

The parathyroid glands are four tiny, rice-grain-sized glands that lie on or within the upper and lower poles of the two lobes of the thyroid. These regulate the amount of calcium in the bloodstream. Too much parathyroid hormone may cause hyperparathyroidism, which may be manifested by calcium kidney stones and gastrointestinal problems, due to elevated blood calcium. Often mild blood calcium elevations are discovered serendipitously when a routine blood chemistry panel is performed. Asymptomatic hyperparathyroidism is more common than previously realized, and many such patients may simply be watched over for a period of time, without ever requiring surgery. Hyperparathyroidism is usually caused by a tumor of one of the parathyroid glands, which almost always is benign. It is readily cured by removal, although locating it may be a problem. Skilled medical and surgical help is necessary. Low parathyroid states may occur after thyroid surgery if the glands are removed or destroyed by the procedure. This sometimes is impossible to avoid. Treatment for low calcium must be given to prevent tetany, a muscular twitching. Calcium taken with vitamin D controls the situation.

Pancreas

The pancreas is a large structure lying deep within the abdomen adjacent to the stomach, liver, and spleen. It is actually two distinct glands. One is exocrine; that is, it makes enzymes that flow into the intestinal tract via canals called the pancreatic ducts. These are digestive enzyme juices, and include amylase for sugar and lipase for fat. Without these chemicals which are secreted when we eat, we could not digest food. We will discuss this later in the gastrointestinal section.

The endocrine pancreas is made up of clusters of special glandular cells located throughout the pancreas. These are called the islets of Langerhans (Langerhans discovered them). These specialized cells produce two important hormones; one is insulin, which gets glucose from the blood into the cells of the body for energy metabolism and storage. A second hormone, glucagon, is secreted when the blood sugar level falls. It tells the liver to release stored glucose into the blood to prevent too low a blood sugar (hypoglycemia), a dangerous condition. We need glucose at all times for energy and brain function. Insulin production has as its primary stimulator a rising level of glucose in the blood. If the pancreas's islets are destroyed and cannot make insulin, the disease known as juvenile diabetes (diabetes mellitus Type 1) occurs. This was invariably fatal until the discovery of insulin by Banting and Best and others in about 1910 to 1915. Diabetes of this type is now managed by insulin injection. In recent years, experts have determined that the closer the blood sugar level is kept to normal, the better the outcome and the healthier the diabetic. In the future it may be possible, via ingenious methods, to provide an artificial pancreas, which may eliminate the considerable time and fuss of testing blood sugar and giving multiple injections which, unfortunately, is currently necessary to get tight control of diabetes.

There is another, more complex, type of diabetes called Type 2. This is the hereditary type, that has a high familial incidence. In this disease the islets of Langerhans and the insulin-producing cells are present, at least in the early stages, and insulin may be present in greater amounts than normal. However, it doesn't seem to get released at the right time and it doesn't work on the cells to get sugar inside at a rapid enough rate. This discovery was made in the 1960s by Drs. Solomon Berson and Rosalind Yalow, for which Yalow won a Nobel prize. (Berson died before he could be so honored.) Incidentally, Banting and Macleod (his boss), won a Nobel prize in 1927 for the discovery of insulin.

Type 2 diabetes is not invariably and rapidly fatal, as used to be the other, juvenile kind. Usually it occurs later in life and often is associated with obesity. It is usually best treated by weight reduction, diet, and regular exercise. This advice is, unhappily, generally not heeded. For one reason or another, most people just can't do it. Other treatments, including medicine of various types taken orally, are helpful in management of Type 2. Insulin injection is usually withheld unless it is absolutely necessary. There have been major advances in oral medication therapy, especially for Type 2 diabetes. Now, frequently, this disease is controllable by use of two or more oral agents rather than advancing to insulin treatment (which has some important disadvantages). In any case, it now appears that tight control of both Types 1 and 2 diabetes does help greatly to prevent complications. It requires some effort but it's worth it. Still, most important are the lifestyle changes mentioned above, which in many cases obviate the need for any medicine.

The major killer of juvenile diabetics is small vessel disease of the arterioles and capillaries, most tragically of the eyes and the kidneys. The great burden of blindness and kidney failure after years of insulin treatment is frequently the lot of the unfortunate juvenile diabetic. It is gratifying to report that with tight control of blood sugar and with other advances in our treatment of these complications, these awful outcomes are somewhat less frequent. The Type 2 diabetic, though also affected by small vessel disease, is usually more troubled by large vessel or arteriosclerotic disease, with the ravages of this disorder (coronary artery disease, stroke, blood vessel closure in the legs) being the most serious complication. This, too, is amenable to modern medical treatment, but it is difficult. Again, it is far better to prevent problems, if at all possible. You can't change your genes, but you can keep yourself and your kids fit and trim, which may be all that is necessary.

Finally, the early symptoms of diabetes should be mentioned. In the juvenile type, the disease usually manifests in a rather dramatic fashion with weight loss, increased thirst, and urination. The blood sugar, being high and unable to get into the cells, is excreted into the urine, thereby increasing the urine flow and water loss. Since, in diabetics, sugar cannot be easily metabolized, stored fat is burned, causing weight loss, and more ominously, acidosis, which is the product of fat metabolism. If the dehydration and acidosis progresses, it may cause the collapse known as diabetic coma. This was the proximate cause of death before the days of insulin, the hormone that prevents these processes.

The adult-onset diabetic has symptoms which are more subtle and may not be evident until serious damage has occurred. The Type 2 diabetic usually does not notice increased thirst and urination until later on, but the metabolic damage may be progressing anyway. Therefore, more adult-onset diabetics are walking around in ignorance of their disease than have been detected. This is another reason for medical visitation in the otherwise seemingly well man. Blood sugar measurements may be the only way this disease is discovered.

Sex Organs

The sex organs (ovaries and testicles) are under the direct and dynamic control of the pituitary and hypothalamus. Clearly, such regular and periodic events as the menstrual cycle require very sophisticated time mechanisms. These "clocks" are situated in the brain and signal appropriately to the hypothalamus and pituitary when and which hormone needs to be released. All this complicated activity has checks and balances, characteristic of the neuroendocrine system. For instance, when a sufficient amount of sex hormone, estrogen in the female and testosterone in the male, is present and active, these hormones in turn tell the pituitary to relax, it's done its job.

The details of the whole process, particularly of the female with her marvelous menstrual and puerperal (reproductive) functioning, are not within the scope of this book, but it behooves us, as men, to understand for our own good. Of course, we have our own endocrine sex life, which will be discussed later.

DR. DASHE'S TIPS FOR HEALTH MAINTENANCE

1. Your glands are meant to work diligently without too much effort on your part. They will only make their presence known to you if something goes wrong.

2. Thyroid problems seem to be more prevalent; although mostly in women, men can have problems as well. Thyroid cancer especially can be easily detected and treated, but you need to give the doctor a chance to find it.

3. If you are a Type 1 diabetic you probably already know it and you are on a regimen of insulin injections. Lifelong maintenance is necessary and many diabetics live long and active lives.

4. Type 2 or adult-onset diabetes is much more common and subtle and also dangerous. If you are obese you might be at risk and will need to take steps to deal with this condition. Often, merely a change in diet and additional exercise will prevent the necessity of medication.

5. Endocrine evaluation is an important part of your physical and routine laboratory examinations.

6. "Male menopause" is still a controversial issue. Treatment with male hormone is available.

7. Use of body-building hormones (steroids) to bulk up, strengthen, or improve performance in athletes, is both illegal and hazardous to your health.

Chapter 10

THE GASTROINTESTINAL SYSTEM

Medical school was, if anything, a desensitizing and broadening experience. I wish it were available to everyone. Professor of Psychiatry Gliebe (pronounced glee-bee) was an astonishing teacher. My first meeting with him was at the San Francisco County Hospital Mental Ward; he was the director and the chief of service. He was a dour, yet elfin, owlish-looking man who had a wry, sharp intelligence. I felt that he was looking at each of us junior medical students (known as clinical clerks) and assessing us with a frosty discernment that made us shiver as we awaited his Olympian words. This, it seemed, was a man who knew everything about us (especially me). Blandly noting our discomfiture, he smiled and said softly and disarmingly, "You know, a good s— is better than a bad f—, anytime!"

This was, as you can imagine, a flabbergasting statement, especially to a twenty-two-year-old naïf like me. The profundity of these coarse and academically taboo words dawned upon me gradually. I have come to call them Gliebe's first law of relativity, expressing as they do in Celtic terms the majestic concept of priority in biology.

It is true. First things must come first. Starvation breeds impotence and sterility. Constipation narrows one's concentration. The gastrointestinal supersedes the genital, and is superseded only by life itself; heart and lungs, breathing and pumping blood.

Anatomy and Physiology

The digestive tract starts out as a simple tube and ends up as a tube with a bunch of twists. Since it is about 22 feet long, from mouth to anus, some curvature is to be expected to cram it all into a limited space. Basically, however, the tube system works well with fuel (food and water) entering and residue leaving with regularity. Any long-term disruption of this pathway is intolerable, usually painful, always embarrassing to say the least, and at worst potentially fatal. The causes and management of such disruptions, at least the most common ones, will be discussed later. First, however, we must mention this food-processing system and the mechanisms involved in its functioning.

Figure 10-1 is a simplified diagram of the parts. The mouth begins coarse processing of ingested food by chewing. Chewed food is propelled down the swallowing tube (esophagus) by muscular contractions known as peristalsis. These waves of contraction are always, in health, propelling contents downward throughout the entire tube, esophagus to rectum. The stomach, a large sac into which the esophagus delivers the chewed meal, is a medium processor. Its digestive juices, pepsin, and hydrochloric acid help break up and dissolve tough bunches, especially muscle fibers of meat. (Why doesn't it digest itself? We'll discuss this in a while.) After stomach processing, the dissolved food is then sent, in jets, through the pyloric valve, into the first part of the small intestine, where major digestion and absorption, with the help of the liver and pancreas, take place. The downward journey is further aided by the presence of one-way valves at key intervals (between the esophagus and stomach, called the cardiac valve because of its proximity to the heart; the gastroduodenal or pyloric valve between the stomach and small intestine; and the ileocolic valve between the small and large

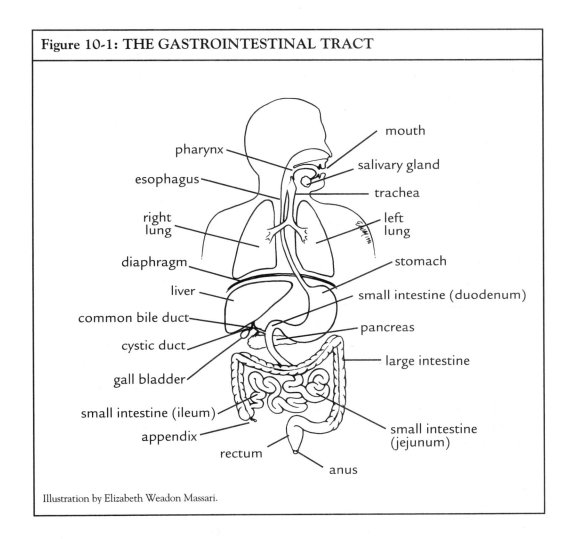

Figure 10-1: THE GASTROINTESTINAL TRACT

Illustration by Elizabeth Weadon Massari.

intestine). Reversal of peristalsis will cause cramps, nausea, and vomiting. All along the tube, various digestive juices are injected to accomplish the goal of the gastrointestinal (GI) tract. Enzymes process and dissolve foods; ptyalin and amylase for sugar, bile acid and lipase for fat, and hydrochloric acid (only in the stomach) and proteases for proteins. The motion and chemicals mix and churn the food and break it up so that absorption may take place, primarily in the small intestine. The processed material, which is liquid by the time it passes through to the colon, is then dehydrated in this large intestine, where water is the main substance absorbed back into the body. The colonic peristalsis finally deposits the semisolid wastes, known as feces, into the end of the tube, the rectum, from which finally it is expelled, completing the journey. All this takes place usually within twenty-four hours, when all is working well.

The liver, which is a large organ in the upper abdomen, is considered a part of the GI system, although it has many other functions as well. For instance, it is a marvelous filter of blood. The food that is absorbed from the GI tract is delivered immediately to the liver via the blood system of the intestinal organs. This system is known as the portal circulation and is entirely separate from the other circulation. Portal blood, carrying dissolved and digested foods such as sugar, amino acids from protein breakdown, and fatty acids from fat digestion, goes to the liver for further processing, storage, and chemical conversion to necessary body chemicals. All blood eventually flows through the liver, where many waste products are removed and excreted into the bile. This is then carried to the gallbladder for storage. Chemicals known as bile acids are formed in the liver and also become part of the bile liquid. These chemicals are necessary to help the digestion of fats, as mentioned above. Bile also contains yellow and green pigments which are derived from the breakdown of hemoglobin from used-up red blood cells, also filtered out by the liver. Finally, the liver is a great chemical factory that is able to remove toxic waste products from the blood; it detoxifies them and also secretes them into bile. This complex bile solution containing these various substances will eventually be injected into the intestinal tract where the digestive substances will work and the waste substances will be excreted into the stool for external disposal.

The gallbladder is simply a storage sac. If it becomes diseased, it can be removed without serious harm to the system.

I have previously described the pancreas as an endocrine gland, making insulin for sugar metabolism. The tissue of the pancreas that is not endocrine is known as the exocrine pancreas, which is by volume the greater portion of the gland and functions separately from the endocrine pancreas. The exocrine pancreas manufactures powerful digestive enzymes which are critical in the digestion and absorption of sugar (amylase) and fat (lipase). These and other enzymes are secreted into the pancreatic duct, which usually joins the common bile duct of the liver. When food enters the stomach and upper small intestine (duodenum), signals are released which cause the gallbladder to contract and the proper valves to relax so that the digestive juices are injected in a timely fashion into the food stream of the small intestine.

The small intestine, which takes up the largest length of the tube, does much of the churning, mixing, digesting, and absorbing of the food. Abnormalities of the small intestine may lead to impaired absorption of food and malnutrition, known as malabsorption.

The colon serves primarily as a dehydrator of liquid material as well as a storage facility. It is a very large looping structure which starts in the right lower abdomen, rises up to the liver in the right upper abdomen, makes a sharp leftward turn under the diaphragm on the left (it is now actually in the chest, right underneath the left side of the heart), and finally takes a twisting, sharp dive downward on the left side of the abdomen over the pelvic brim into the pelvis where it ends in the rectum. It is a ride like a roller coaster, which explains why crampy gas bubbles in the colon can be felt all over the abdomen, even in the chest (where they can be mistaken for heart pain).

The rectum and anus are the end of the line but are just as important as any other GI structures. Without proper functioning of these organs, our society would probably be primitive and intolerable by current standards. The rectum tells us when we need to defecate and, after toilet training, permits us to choose the time and place. The anal sphincter has the uncanny ability to distinguish between solid, liquid, and gas and to permit us to release them and, if we demand, to hold it in.

Common Diseases of the Gastrointestinal Tract

Mouth

We don't usually think of the mouth as part of this system, even though it initiates the gastrointestinal journey. Many other functions are assumed by this complex opening, but biting and chewing food efficiently is a high priority. For this reason, I advise periodic dental consultation and care. You should be aware of the dangers of oral tobacco products, both chewing tobacco and snuff. There is little question about the relation of this form of tobacco usage with disease, both benign and malignant (ask your dentist about tooth and gum loss). Cancer of the mouth, throat, and esophagus occur with such regularity in tobacco chewers (smokers too) that even baseball players are no longer permitted to "chew." Bubble gum seems to be an acceptable substitute (but not in time to save Babe Ruth and Brett Butler from mouth and throat cancer).

The digestive glands of the mouth are known as the salivary glands (parotid, submaxillary, and submental). The glands make saliva, which is a complex liquid substance that seems to have minor antiseptic and digestive functions (ptyalin, a saliva enzyme, breaks complex sugars down to glucose), but mainly is a lubricant to help the chewed food easily slide down the esophagus to the stomach. Salivary glands may be subject to infection (mumps parotitis) or tumors.

Esophagus

The esophagus is an interesting and very important organ. It conducts food from the pharynx down to the stomach through the cardiac valve. This valve is extremely important. When it malfunctions it can cause serious troubles, such as the inability to swallow when it is stuck closed by a muscle spasm or stricture. This is a frightening and most uncomfortable condition and needs to be treated promptly by a gastroenterologist. The obstruction may be quickly relieved by use of a flexible endoscope (fiberoptic tube). Prevention of recurrence by various means is usually quite successful. Closure of the tube by a tumor (almost always malignant) is a terrible disease, again most often related to tobacco use. Surgery can usually be done for relief after the diagnosis is made, but the prognosis is generally grim.

Far more common is the condition known as gastroesophageal reflux disease (GERD). All of us, at one time or another, have experienced the symptom of heartburn. This lower chest discomfort, sometimes associated with overeating, belching, and a sour taste in the back of the throat, is usually caused by dietary indiscretion. An overly distended stomach sends its acidic contents back into the esophagus up through the cardiac valve. The lining of the esophagus is not prepared to accept this backup. For one thing, stomach juice is highly acidic (hydrochloric acid, the same stuff used in swimming pools, is an extremely strong acid). The esophagus is designed for a neutral, neither acid nor alkaline, content. Acid from the stomach or the strong alkali from further down (bile is alkaline) causes irritation and an uncomfortable burning sensation in the chest. Antacids, such as calcium carbonate (Tums) or magnesium and aluminum salts (Maalox) usually offer rapid relief. I have found that Gaviscon, which floats on top of the stomach contents and bathes the lower esophageal area as well, helps a lot, particularly at night after retiring. Reclining aggravates the situation because gravity works against peristalsis to abet the backward flow.

A word regarding the term *hiatus hernia*. The hiatus is the hole in the diaphragm where the esophagus and the stomach join. This space is generally snug enough to act as a support to the esophagus-stomach valve (cardiac valve) junction. When the diaphragmatic hole is overstretched, the stomach may herniate, or project upward into the chest, either temporarily or permanently. It was once thought that this caused constant valve failure; that stomach contents would always flow backward into the esophagus. This does not always seem to happen. Many people may have hiatus hernia with little or no backflow (reflux is the medical term). Chronic valve failure, when it cannot close adequately much or all of the time, gives rise to the more serious GERD syndrome, where esophageal inflammation or ulceration may take place. Occasionally GERD may be associated with respiratory symptoms. This happens when stomach contents are aspirated into the trachea at night, when the patient is asleep and unaware that this is happening. It may be the cause of sudden onset of nocturnal asthma in an older (usually overweight) person. Chronic GERD may lead to scarring of the lower esophagus with partial blockage of the tube, which may require mechanical stretching. Some experts think that it also may lead to precancerous changes (Barrett's esophagus) and eventually cancer if not detected and treated.

Treatment of GERD is somewhat controversial. For the minor, transient occurrence, use of antacids and avoidance of overdoing the amount and fat content of meals may be all that is necessary. Weight reduction, of any amount, is helpful. Frequent recurrence or regular discomfort warrants further investigation and treatment. Endoscopy may be called for, wherein a specialist (usually a gastroenterologist) visualizes the upper GI tract through a flexible fiberoptic tube about ⅜ of an inch wide. The doctor can determine whether serious disease exists in the lower esophagus. If so, appropriate strong measures may be prescribed. Medications used include acid-formation blockers such as omeprazole. Other useful drugs, such as cisapride, speed stomach emptying and help tighten the cardiac sphincter valve. Weight loss and propping up the head of the bed about 6 inches may also be effective in decreasing acid reflux during the night. Some experts, particularly surgeons, feel strongly that serious GERD should be treated with surgery and that medical treatment is merely a stopgap measure. They believe that a procedure known as fundoplication, or building up and strengthening the area of the gastroesophageal valve (thus restoring its valvular function), is the only proper treatment. This even may be done, in experienced hands, via "keyhole surgery" techniques requiring only a few tiny abdominal incisions, using microsurgical methods. It sounds good, but the matter is far from settled, particularly since regular use of omeprazole seems safe and effective, even on a long-term basis.

Stomach and Duodenum

Ulcers (peptic ulcer disease). The stomach has not only the ability to manufacture hydrochloric acid but also, amazingly, resistance to its caustic action. The stomach also manufactures pepsin, another protein-breaking enzyme. The combination of hydrochloric acid and pepsin is strong enough to turn a piece of tough steak into a liquid puddle. So why doesn't the stomach attack and absorb itself? We don't know for sure. We know that mucus produced by the stomach lining is protective and so is the gut hormone, prostaglandin. Acid and pepsin production is stimulated by eating. The central nervous system via the vagus nerve, which goes to the stomach, and the hormone gastrin, send the message that food is present. Chemicals such as alcohol, nicotine, and histamine are direct stimulators of acid secretion. Stress may itself be an acid-producing factor, although experts no longer accept that this is the major cause of peptic ulcer.

Drugs, notably aspirin and other non-steroidal anti-inflammatory agents (known as NSAIDs), may contribute to ulcer formation by being irritants in themselves, thereby injuring the lining of the gut, and also by having a strong antiprosta-glandin effect as part of their anti-inflammatory activity. It is hoped that the new COX-2 inhibitor type NSAIDs (Celebrex and Vioxx®) will avert this potentially serious complication. Peptic ulceration may occur in any area that stomach contents touch, including the esophagus (about 5 percent), the stomach itself (about 5 percent) and the most common place for ulceration, the first part of the small intestine, just south of the pyloric valve, the area known as the duodenum (90 percent). The duodenum is not protected from an acid environment as is the stomach, and any amount of acid sent its way can cause an ulcer. Presence of acid is necessary for peptic ulcer production. Ulcers that appear anyplace in the upper gastrointestinal tube in the absence of acid must be due to something else, such as a tumor or other damage (as from NSAIDs). It is a particular concern when stomach ulcers are present in the absence of acid production. If complete healing is not seen (by x-ray or direct observation through the gastroscope) within three weeks of treatment, biopsy is warranted, because often this type of ulcer is due to stomach cancer. Peptic ulcers are extremely common, occurring in as much as 10 percent of the population. The disease is twice as common in men as in women and usually occurs in people between the ages of forty-five and sixty-five. We don't know why. What about the good old scapegoat, stress? A recent discovery is of major importance. Researchers have found a peculiar bacteria called *Helicobacter pylori* in association with an extremely high number of cases of peptic ulcer (up to 90 percent). Not only is the germ associated but, if eradicated by appropriate intensive antibiotic treatment, the ulcer is cured and recurrences infrequent. This astounding finding seems to have withstood all scientific attack and, although the concept of an infectious cause of peptic ulcer had long ago been postulated (during the days of Pasteur and Koch, just about all disease was thought to be infectious) and rejected, it has now been accepted as a proven phenomenon and the treatment promulgated.

Acid, however, is still an important part of the story. Successful *H. pylori* treatment requires intensive anti-acid therapy as well as antibiotics. The bacteria either requires or causes overproduction of acid to do its dirty work. The diagnosis of *H. pylori* infection is still in the process of development and methods range from stomach biopsy through an endoscope and various blood tests to a simple noninvasive breath test (called ^{13}C-urea). The breath test will probably become the standard, since a positive test denotes a current active infection.

Symptoms of peptic ulcer disease vary, but typically ulcers manifest themselves by a deep, aching, hungerlike pain in the midupper abdomen that is rapidly relieved by eating food or taking an antacid. Often the pain awakens one during the night or may be present as a severe hunger pang an hour or two after eating. The pain may have a burning or penetrating quality, but is usually only mild to moderate. Aspirin, coffee, or alcohol aggravates it, and antacid relief is common. When it occurs, it suggests the diagnosis. Complications of ulcers are now relatively rare because of our newer treatments but include obstruction, perforation, and bleeding in the GI tract. Obstruction usually occurs after chronic or recurrent disease with scarring and closing down of the scar. (I haven't seen this happen for years.) Actual perforation of an ulcer through the wall of the stomach or duodenum is also rare; when it occurs, it is a violent life-threatening situation requiring immediate surgery. The patient is usually in shock with intense, sudden, severe abdominal pain. Surgical exploration is obviously indicated. In my experience, the most common complication is that of massive ulcer bleeding. This seems, these days, to be caused almost always by the prior use of aspirin or other nonsteroid anti-inflammatory drugs (NSAIDs). It is frequently painless, probably because blood itself acts as an antacid. Bloody vomiting, although rare, spectacularly announces the diagnosis. Far more common is simple weakness, fainting upon arising, and tarry black bowel movements (acid turns blood into a sticky, tarry mass).

Confirmation of a peptic ulcer was usually done via upper gastrointestinal x-ray using liquid barium swallows to outline and locate the ulcer crater. Although this still is an excellent technique, it has been superseded by endoscopy, which is quick, relatively painless with the flexible fiberoptic scopes, and may be done at the patient's bedside, a particularly valuable technique for situations where there is bleeding or when the patient is very sick.

Most peptic ulcers are easily and rapidly treated at home with the medicines now available. Forty years ago we were limited to antacids, rest, and diet. The so-called "Sippy diet" (after a doctor named Sippy), was half and half (milk and cream), alternating with antacids, every thirty minutes to an hour, day and night. This was used for the worst cases. Today, much has changed. For one thing, diets are hardly restricted at all, except for hard-to-digest foods, alcohol, and irritating medicines. Also, we have a choice of highly effective anti-acid medications, especially the so-called H2 blockers (histamine, type 2 receptor antagonists), including cimetadine (Tagamet), ranitidine (Zantac), famotidine (Pepcid), and others that have proven remarkably effective in both treatment and prevention of ulcer recurrence. These drugs, which act in six to twenty-four hours, have revolutionized treatment in the past twenty years. Even stronger medicines are the acid-pump blockers such as omeprazole (Prilosec®) and lansoprazole (Prevacid®), which stop acid production totally and will heal any peptic ulcer that the H2 blockers can't. Antacids of the various types previously mentioned remain useful, particularly if taken often enough (which is sometimes hard to do). They have taken a backseat to these newer acid-preventing drugs, especially since some of the latter have become available over the counter (Tagamet, Zantac, and Pepcid), and are, therefore, more economical.

Surgery for peptic ulcer disease has become, for the most part, a thing of the past. Partial stomach removal is rarely done and is actually not as effective as are medical treatments. Surgery is pretty much restricted to treatment of perforated ulcers and the rare cases of obstruction or persistent bleeding.

Dyspepsia. This is a general term meaning upper abdominal discomfort, usually after eating. It is commonly due to the indiscreet ingestion of food by type (too fatty) or amount (too much), but occasionally it may signify a more severe gastrointestinal problem, such as peptic ulcer or gallbladder, liver, or pancreatic inflammation. So if discomfort is very severe or persistent, evaluation and examination by your doctor is necessary. "Nervous stomach" is a common problem, but I am never quite content with this diagnosis unless other illness is excluded by careful history, physical examination, and if warranted, laboratory and x-ray studies. Assuming any psychosomatic diagnosis is, in my opinion, bad medicine. A personal physician is in an advantageous position here. There is nothing as helpful in diagnosis as seeing a patient over a long period of time. Subtle changes in health status may become evident this way. It is better by far to be a doctor who has the ability to observe a patient over time than a brilliant professor-type who has to know everything in fifteen minutes—this usually can't be done.

Liver, Pancreas, and Gallbladder

There are too many possible afflictions of these gastrointestinal adjunctive organs to discuss all of them at length. I shall mention the ones of greatest frequency and importance for the informed patient, which is what I want you to be.

Liver

Hepatitis. The liver is so incredibly important that it deserves an encyclopedia rather than a paragraph. But since I must limit my discussion, I choose to emphasize the subject of hepatitis. The most common cause of this inflammatory disease is viral. Over the past fifty years researchers have determined that there are many viruses that can affect the liver. These viruses have been identified by letters (I believe we are up to G). The most prevalent ones are types A, B, and C, which are also the only ones regularly detected by routine laboratory means. These nasty and unpredictable germs can either lay you low, kill you, or leave you blissfully unaware of their presence, depending upon your native resistance and luck. In my own case, it was determined by laboratory testing, after I had stuck myself with a needle from an alleged hepatitis carrier, that I have antibodies to hepatitis B in my bloodstream. I must have gotten it sometime in my past medical career, although I didn't know it.

Hepatitis A, or the epidemic type, is the kind one gets from ingesting contaminated food and water that is handled by an infected individual; you can get it from your local hamburger house, taco stand, or fancy restaurant. Hepatitis B also may be disseminated via the oral route but, of greater importance, may be transmitted by semen and by blood (via drug needles or transfusion). Hepatitis C seems to be strictly blood borne. Now that we have tests for this (and hepatitis B) at blood donor sites, donor blood is safer and transfusion hepatitis is less frequent. The other viral types that are not easily detected may be present in donor blood so it is best, by far, to avoid blood transfusion, if possible, or to self-donate blood if elective surgery is scheduled.

There are now good vaccines available for hepatitis A and B. All children should be immunized, I believe. For now, hepatitis immunization is available and advisable for those at high risk (health workers, foreign travelers).

Cirrhosis. This liver disease is due to inflammation followed by severe scarring of the liver tissue, usually caused by viral infection or toxic chemicals. Cirrhosis, although seemingly less frequent these days, still occurs and is a major killer of habitual drinkers. Other liver toxins include cleaning fluids, benzene, poisonous mushrooms, and certain drugs. Acetaminophen (Tylenol) in large doses, and especially when combined with alcohol, is an example of a substance that can cause severe drug-induced liver toxicity. It's far better to keep your own liver than to try to get a transplant, so take good care of it.

Gallbladder

This storage sac, located under the liver (see Figure 10-1), causes more trouble than it's worth. The reason for this statement is that we seemingly don't need gallbladders. People appear to get along perfectly well without one. This bile storage container has the unfortunate propensity to develop the oysterlike habit of forming pearls, which are called gallstones. Bile is the liquid secreted by the liver and stored in the gallbladder for use in digestion. It seems to be unstable and sometimes forms these solid concretions, known as calculi, which can on occasion travel up the bile ducts and obstruct them. This obstruction causes severe pain and inflammation, and often infection including gangrene. Occasionally, gangrene of the gallbladder may result in a surgical emergency. More frequently, the pain is episodic and transient. Recurrent or sporadic gallbladder attacks may occur with or without warning. A fatty meal is a common provocation. Gallstones may be present and asymptomatic throughout a person's life, so controversy exists regarding the necessity of action in asymptomatic individuals. Surgeons generally favor the removal of the organ (no surprise) for reasons that are not without merit; one never knows when an attack will happen. Gallstones may cause gallbladder cancer from chronic irritation (a very rare cancer). It is now easier to remove the gallbladder through the keyhole microscopic endo-scopic technique. My feeling is that if it isn't causing problems, don't do it. Occasionally a gallstone may escape into and obstruct the common bile duct (Figure 10-1) and block the flow of bile entirely from the liver to the intestine. This is a serious situation requiring surgical intervention. The blockage and backup of bile causes jaundice (bile pigment buildup in the blood) which stains the skin and eyes yellow-green. Jaundice is also a feature of liver disease when the liver cannot function well enough to excrete bile into the bile ducts.

Pancreas

The pancreas may also be affected by obstruction of the common bile duct. If the pancreatic duct is also involved, bile may flow into the pancreas and activate the potent pancreatic enzymes, which may start digesting the pancreas itself. This is called acute pancreatitis and is a most painful and dangerous disease. Pancreatitis may occur without gallstone obstruction. This usually is related to malnutrition and/or alcoholism and high blood triglycerides. In any case, pancreatitis requires skillful hospital care for treatment. If pancreas damage is severe enough, chronic pancreatitis with digestive consequences may ensue. This includes chronic diar-rhea and malnutrition due to the inability to digest foods properly. This is called malabsorption. Pancreas enzymes can be taken by mouth, which may be of some help. Cancer of the pancreas is the most frequently missed cancer because of its hidden location, way back in the abdomen touching the spine. When it is symp-tomatic (the usual complaint is mysterious back pain), it is usually incurable. Total removal is almost impossible. Some chemotherapy may be promising. There is no known cause.

The Small Bowel (Midgut)

This part of the tube is the longest (approximately 12 feet) and, though men-tioned least, plays a vital nutritional role, absorbing food after it's been "lopped and chopped" above. When the small bowel doesn't function, you don't absorb food, so it's as if you don't eat. Fortunately, this area is not subject to problems as frequently as its northern and southern neighbors. Any interruption in function, however, will prove very disastrous. There aren't too many serious disorders of the small bowel, other than the above-mentioned duodenal ulcer (the duodenum, jejunum, and ileum are the three parts of the midgut). Crohn's disease (regional ileitis or enteritis) got a few headlines in the fifties and sixties because of former President Eisenhower's illness, and indeed it is a serious problem. It is categorized as one of the inflammatory bowel diseases (IBD) and, along with ulcerative colitis, is a major gastrointestinal disorder often requiring intense treatment and surgical intervention.

There are some interesting and strange small bowel absorption disorders known as sprue. One variety, seen in temperate countries, is thought to be a manifestation of allergy to gluten, a wheat protein. Tropical sprue is probably caused by a virus, or other infection, as yet unidentified.

The Large Bowel

It may be last, but it is not least. For most of us, the day begins with a visit to the bathroom to empty the bladder. The kidneys have filtered and cleansed our blood overnight and have sent the soluble waste products down to the bladder for elimination. The morning pee must be taken care of promptly, and we know it in no uncertain terms. It is not the same, however, for the solid waste disposal system—the large bowel. Morning emptying does not automatically occur for several reasons. First, colonic peristalsis must be awakened. Second, the colon, obliging organ that it is, will retain feces for later disposal, if asked to do so. It is, unfortunately, asked far too often.

Colonic movement is initiated from above. Peristalsis, as you recall, goes from north to south or from front to end of the gastrointestinal tube. Therefore, the process of defecation is usually started by eating or drinking something. That morning cup of coffee or other hot liquid is a prime mover. Eating a full breakfast has become a thing of the past for most of us, and even taking the time to initiate peristalsis conveniently seems to have become a luxury in Western civilization. This is the direct cause of the most common disorder of the large bowel, functional constipation (sometimes called "commuters' constipation"). This latter-day adult toilet mistraining has caused much misery. I have made many people happy by telling them to arise fifteen minutes earlier, and have a cup of coffee or tea or hot water, and take some pleasant reading into the loo, be seated, and just wait for the epiphany. As Professor Louis Armstrong said, "Leave all your troubles behind you."

Constipation is not simply a matter of lack of frequency of bowel movements. It really means difficulty with defecation, usually due to hard and dried-out stools. This happens because the colon absorbs water as its major function. Stools that are not timely eliminated are sent back up for further processing, which means further drying. There are other causes of constipation, such as acute dehydration, weakening illnesses, hypothyroidism, neurologic disease, and so on. All require professional evaluation and treatment. Occasionally, one can handle simple constipation, if not an ongoing problem requiring such evaluation, by judicious and occasional use of a laxative (see chapter 4, "When to Call a Doctor"). If there is great discomfort and immediate action is desired, a suppository, either the glycerine type or stronger (Dulcolax®), or an enema, such as the convenient low-volume disposable type (Fleet® enema), may be used. This should be a rare event. It is far better to maintain regularity with good toilet habits, as described above, and a healthy diet. Regular intake of high-fiber foods (roughage, a truly natural laxative) not only tends to lower blood cholesterol, but is associated with lower incidences of colon, breast, and other cancers, and is stimulatory to the large bowel.

Diarrheal diseases. There are too many of these to detail at length but the common and transient ones usually respond promptly to simple measures. The violence of the process as well as the response to mild remedies and the persistence of the problem determine the timing, if necessary, of seeking medical care. Bloody diarrhea, rapid dehydration with attendant weakness and faintness, or severe abdominal pain require immediate attention. Milder cases usually respond to a low residue diet, limited to tea, water, Gatorade® or other electrolyte drinks, steamed rice, apple juice, apple sauce, banana, white meat of poultry, and bouillon; and the use of Pepto-Bismol (1 tablespoon every hour or two; don't forget Pepto-Bismol may turn everything black, including the tongue and the toilet) and, if necessary, bowel relaxers such as Lomotil or Imodium. In any case, if diarrhea persists much longer than one week, a visit to the doctor is in order. What is worrisome in such cases is not so much the infectious diarrheas (dysenteries) but the more onerous inflammatory bowel diseases such as ulcerative colitis and regional enteritis (Crohn's disease). Also, occasionally an unsuspected bowel cancer presents itself as chronic diarrhea.

Irritable bowel syndrome. For some reason, this is far more common in women than in men. Some suggest, but have not proven, that it is a psychosomatic disorder, perhaps a response to chronic emotional stress. It is the common final diagnosis when the doctor has excluded other causes of alternating constipation and diarrhea and chronic abdominal cramping and discomfort. I have never, as a physician, been comfortable with simply blaming this on emotions. I strongly believe that a patient with such complaints deserves a complete history and thorough evaluation, usually to include lower bowel endoscopy (colonoscopy or flexible sigmoidoscopy) and barium enema x-ray. If examination excludes structural disease, irritable bowel syndrome is probably the correct diagnosis. The treatment should be symptomatic and sympathetic, and not judgmental.

Inflammatory bowel diseases. Ulcerative colitis and regional enteritis are usually marked by persistent and uncontrollable diarrhea, frequently with blood-tinged or streaked stools. It is also frequently associated with weight loss, malaise, and other physical symptoms such as joint aches. Inflammatory bowel disease is often a difficult problem that requires lifelong treatment and observation. This is best done by a gastroenterology specialist. Much research has been and is being done to better the lives and comfort of such patients; the outlook is far better than it used to be.

Appendicitis. The vermiform (wormlike) appendix is a small, hollow appendage of the cecal (right side) part of the colon (Figure 10-1). Presumably it is a vestige of an extra part of the gastrointestinal tract that was utilized in ancient man for digestion of vegetable matter. Other vegetarian mammals have much larger appendices for this purpose. Now the appendix seems to have no better purpose than to provide surgical practice to my scalpel-wielding colleagues. When the appendix becomes blocked or infected, it may burst (perforate) and cause peritonitis. The symptoms begin with severe abdominal pain, and progress to pain localized to the right side of the lower abdomen.

Diverticulosis and diverticulitis. Diverticuli of the colon are small pouches that develop in the colon wall, usually on the left side. These small herniations may be due to inborn weakness of spots in the colon wall, or increased pressure within the colon, or both. They seem to occur more often in individuals who have bowel problems such as dysfunctional constipation or irritable bowel syndrome, but this has not been documented. In any case, having diverticuli is not a disease unless, as in appendicitis, they become obstructed and infected. This latter complication may be very serious and may become a surgical emergency. Perforation of the bowel can result, creating peritonitis and abscess formation in the abdomen. The illness usually appears as a combination of pain, tenderness (particularly in the left lower abdomen), and fever. Occasionally lower gastrointestinal bleeding may arise from a diverticulum. Quick medical attention is vital. Perforation is caused by breakdown of the wall of the diverticulum, and peritonitis may be averted by prompt antibiotic treatment. Appendicitis behaves similarly, only the pain and tenderness is usually on the right side of the abdomen.

Gas. Politely known as flatus, this ubiquitous and embarrassing lower gastrointestinal product has served as a source of much amusement. Professor Walter Alvarez was the great student of flatus. At the University of California, my alma mater, he was the professor of medicine and gastroenterology. He later moved onward and upward to the Mayo Clinic and was a hugely successful medical syndicated columnist for many major national newspapers. His clinical research was legendary at UC. His subjects were financially strapped medical students. He paid his subjects as much as a dollar per day for several classic studies. The first one consisted of stuffing sterile cotton up the rectum to simulate constipation to see what simple colonic distention would do, symptomatically. The answer came quickly. Such distention produced the symptoms generally ascribed to auto-intoxication; malaise, weakness, depression, loss of enthusiasm for life, and a worried expression, all of which disappeared promptly with cotton removal. Alvarez then did the definitive study on bowel gas. He inserted balloon rectal catheters into the student volunteers and measured gas output over a period of several days. Rate and volume of production were carefully monitored and the gas analyzed chemically. The results were truly enlightening. The students, who were not chosen particularly for known lepetomania (excessive flatus production), put out an almost constant flow of gas, amounting to between 20 and 50 liters per day. Most of the gas was nitrogen, air that had been swallowed! Nitrogen cannot be absorbed into the body by the gastrointestinal tract. All that is swallowed must be eliminated below. Gum chewers had much greater output, as did nervous gulpers. The more malodorous bacterial hydrogen sulfide and other bacteria-generated hydrocarbons (the large bowel is inhabited by a rich variety of bacteria living in peace with us that are actually useful in some ways) are a small fraction of the total production. This proved that in the healthy human, flatulence is the normal condition, and, therefore, is not a disease. It does occasionally call for management. Air swallowers beware, especially gum chewers. Certain foods, particularly beans and some leguminous vegetables, are gas-bacteria delicacies and one should avoid them if prone to too much gas production. Beano®, a starch-breaking enzyme, may help. As noted above, lepetomania is excessive flatus production. Monsieur LePetomane (a stage name; his real name was Francis Pujol) was a legendary, celebrated turn-of-the-century concert flatus-flautist (flutist). Please believe this. I could not have made it up. He regaled the capitals of fin-de-siecle Europe with his stirring renditions of Offenbach, Wagner, Verdi and, for le grand finale, "La Marseillaise."

Hemorrhoids. This is one of the few diseases named after an anatomical structure. The rectum and anus, as all other parts of the body, are supplied with arteries and veins, which are called the hemorrhoidal vessels. There are two sets: internal, which supply the rectum, and external, which supply the anus. The distinction is important because hemorrhoids (or "piles"), which are actually nothing other than varicose (blown-out and distended) veins, have different manifestations and symptoms depending upon whether they are the internal (rectal) or external (anal) type. External piles usually bother a person by developing a clot which appears suddenly and painfully at the anus, where it can be felt as a tender lump. Your mirror or loved one will tell you that it looks like a blue grape! It is generally frightening (except to the doctor) because the immediate thought is *cancer*. It isn't. Actually it goes away, usually within a week or so, even if nothing is done. I usually recommend a low-residue diet (no pits or bran), a stool softener, and sitz baths (sitting in a tub of warm water). If the pain is severe, a simple office procedure of slitting the lump and popping out the clot (sounds horrible but it isn't), brings immediate relief. Incidentally, predisposition to hemorrhoids of both types is probably an inherited trait (as are varicose veins of the legs), but they are often precipitated by actions that increase blood pressure in the hemorrhoidal veins, such as straining at bowel movements (constipation or diarrhea), sitting on the toilet for long periods, and standing motionless for hours on end. Preparation H® and similar preparations probably add nothing to the treatment except for some soothing lubrication, but they can't hurt.

Internal hemorrhoids are a more serious problem. They don't hurt but they bleed, sometimes a lot. Severe anemia may develop if the bleeding is not controlled. Hard stools passing through the rectum may easily tear or bruise the veins, causing the bleeding. The internal hemorrhoidal veins are connected to the portal (or liver) blood circulation, so that any liver congestion, such as cirrhosis or alcoholism, may contribute to internal hemorrhoidal bleeding. If internal hemorrhoids cannot be controlled by simple measures (diet, stool softeners, avoidance of constipation or diarrhea), proctologic intervention may be required. Internal piles may respond to office measures including freezing or cautery, but occasionally surgical removal is necessary, particularly if they are so large that they prolapse through the anus and must be constantly pushed back in.

Rectal bleeding may be, and usually is, caused by such benign disease such as hemorrhoids, fissures, or ano-rectal irritation, but it is a matter that deserves further investigation. There can be more serious problems, discussed below:

Polyps or Tumors. Colo-rectal cancers have so increased in frequency that the total number of these in the American population (both male and female) exceeds that of any other single malignancy except the lung. Unfortunately, these are sneaky tumors and by the time symptoms occur, it is often too late for cure. This has become a particularly knotty problem, for early detection as a public health measure is difficult, expensive, and frequently rejected by the public.

Let me define the problem a bit further. Benign tumors of the colon usually present themselves as polyps, or little outgrowths of the internal colonic lining. They may be flat (*sessile* is the medical term) or on a stalk, resembling a mushroom. Polyps are common and usually benign, although occasionally they have the beginnings of malignancy, when seen on microscopic examination. Unfortunately, they are often premalignant and the only sure way to deal with them is by removing them. Most polyps (and cancers) occur in the portion of the colon nearest to the rectum. Until about twenty years ago, the only ones that could be removed without major abdominal surgery were the ones within reach of a rigid tube known as a sigmoidoscope, its maximum length about 12 inches. The advent of fiberoptics has changed all this, and now instruments of almost any length can be passed through any tube system, bends, curves, and all. Surgeons regularly perform procedures including biopsy, removal, and cautery (with electric current and laser) of polyps or other lesions. The diagnostic use of these marvelous instruments has revolutionized the field of gastroenterology and has made the early detection and treatment of colo-rectal tumors and polyps a relatively simple and practical procedure. (Figure 10-2).

The question is, Who should undergo colonic investigation considering 1) the cost, 2) the discomfort, and 3) the fact that there aren't enough scopes or scopers to investigate everyone? There are two types of lower gastrointestinal endoscopes. A short one, about 40 to 70 centimeters in length (15 to 25 inches), is called a flexible sigmoidoscope and may be used for screening and biopsy. This will detect 50 to 60 percent of colon tumors, since this is the area where the majority originate. The colonoscope, which is about three to four times longer, can reach the entire colon. This examination (called colonoscopy) is far more difficult and must be done by an expert, since twists and curves must be skillfully navigated to avoid perforating the bowel wall. It requires a special operating room with uniquely trained nurses. Mild anesthesia is given. Colonoscopy, therefore, is not a screening procedure. The shorter procedure, called sigmoidoscopy, is simpler and easier for the patient and doctor. Many primary physicians have been trained to do this examination. (Kaiser Permanente, an HMO medical group, has at least one clinic that does many screening sigmoidoscopies utilizing highly trained nurse technicians who do nothing else.)

The American Cancer Society recommends that everyone over the age of forty-five have this procedure done at least once, repeated, if nothing is found, every five years. This is not possible for most people. This is my recommendation to patients, when asked for advice in this matter: First, have an occult blood

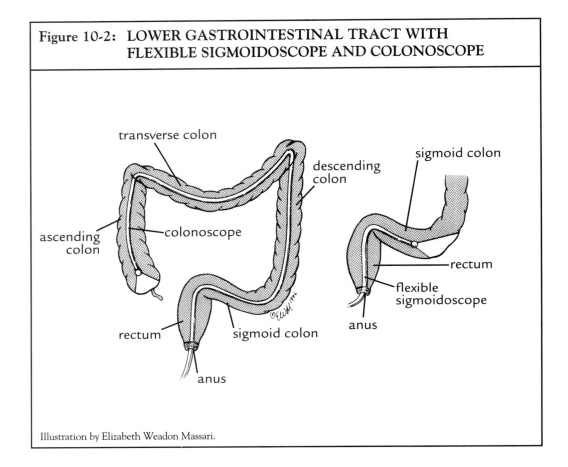

**Figure 10-2: LOWER GASTROINTESTINAL TRACT WITH
FLEXIBLE SIGMOIDOSCOPE AND COLONOSCOPE**

Illustration by Elizabeth Weadon Massari.

stool test every year after the age of thirty-five. This test consists of taking a small sample of three consecutive bowel movements with a little wooden paddle, smearing them on a card provided for the purpose, and mailing it to the doctor for chemical testing. (I have gotten worse mail.) This is inexpensive, not embarrassing, and has been shown to be effective in detecting one of the earliest signs of colon trouble, occult (hidden) blood in the stool. Red meat and some foods have to be avoided for two to three days before the test to prevent false-positive results. Of course, if you have a yearly rectal examination the test can be done then, when the doctor checks the prostate and rectum for abnormality. You really should do this simple test. Then, if the occult blood test is positive, sigmoidoscopy is warranted as well as some other test to detect abnormalities that might be higher in the colon. Usually this is a colon x-ray study (lower GI or barium enema). Full colonoscopy is the alternative, although more costly. There is controversy regarding which is better, but in my opinion, either will suffice.

Who else, other than bleeders, should be screened with sigmoidoscopy? In my judgment there are three other candidate groups: those people who have a family history of colo-rectal cancer, since there is definitely a familial tendency; those who have persistent lower gastrointestinal symptoms such as diarrhea, constipation, or pain; and those who want to have cancer screening no matter what. It's unfortunate, but many people who should do it, just won't.

In summary, the gastrointestinal system, which is responsible for nutrition, thus insuring life itself, takes precedence over many things, including reproductive function.

DR. DASHE'S TIPS FOR HEALTH MAINTENANCE

1. The digestive system is a fuel processing mechanism which is marked by a natural rhythmic propelling action called peristalsis. Obstruction, paralysis, or reversal of flow direction is big trouble.

2. Acid problems, from dyspepsia (heartburn) to ulcers, although temporarily relieved by various antacid medicines, are of many possible causes and frequently require expert diagnosis for proper treatment.

3. Intestinal gas is a general and natural phenomenon, most of it is from swallowed air. Diet can also play a part in the manufacture of gas.

4. Diarrhea and constipation are common problems to all of us and usually require simple steps for control. There are many effective over-the-counter medications available. Be aware that prolonged diarrhea can lead to dehydration, so make sure you get plenty of liquids.

5. Constipation is usually caused by not allowing enough time in the morning to go. Give your gut a break and get up a few minutes earlier.

6. Colon tumors and cancer are exceedingly common, and the incidence is increasing. Early detection is a must for proper treatment, and the means to do so are available but underutilized.

7. Once again, a proper diet that is high in fiber and an active lifestyle will help keep the entire system running smoothly.

8. Hepatitis vaccines are now available. Check with your doctor.

Chapter 11

THE GENITOURINARY SYSTEM

My patients and friends have made it abundantly clear to me that a book about men's health must spend much time "below the belt." As a man I must get down off my pedantic horse and admit that a good portion of my own life has been spent musing about the subject of sexuality, both objectively and otherwise. As a male physician, it is of paramount importance to be aware of one's own feelings and to try to detach them, as much as possible, from one's professional activity.

Well, all this thinking and musing has given me certain insights which I shall share with you. I divide this information into three separate sections: the genitourinary system, anatomy and organ disorders; the prostate and its disorders; and sexual health including functional problems, sexually transmitted diseases, and how to deal with the sexual revolution during this era of AIDS.

Anatomy

The male genitourinary system is both a magnificent and problematic plumbing device (Figures 11-1 and 11-2). Perhaps that's what one can expect from an important dual-functioning apparatus, for that is precisely what it is. First, most important for daily living, is the excretory function. The kidneys, marvelous paired bean-shaped organs that they are, are a deluxe filtration system. The entire blood volume passes through this maze of blood vessels and filtering sacs (known as glomeruli) about 120 times per day. Soluble impurities and end products of metabolism (the ashes of energy burning and cell activity) are selectively removed along with just enough water to keep them dissolved. This creates urine, which is sent down the collecting tubes of the kidneys into the major pipes known as ureters. These ducts are each approximately 12 inches long in the adult. The ureters terminate in the top side of the bladder, where valves are present to prevent backflow into the kidneys when bladder contraction occurs, at the time of urination. The bladder is a muscular balloon which sits right behind the pubic bone in the pelvis. It is capable of expanding to as much as 1½ quarts (1,500 ml) before rupturing (this never happens unless it is somehow severely traumatized). The exit of the bladder is surrounded by a strong smooth muscle (involuntary type) known as the internal sphincter. Just outside of this there is an external sphincter muscle, which is a voluntary one. It's the one you use when you try to "keep it in." The tube leading from the bladder is called the urethra. The first part of the urethra is surrounded by the prostate gland and has tubular connections to the sexual apparatus. Semen enters the plumbing system at this point. The rest of the urethra, known as the penile urethra, is an expandable corrugated tube which leads to the outside of the body (Figure 11-1).

Second, the sexual function of the genitourinary apparatus is, to many of us and to nature as well, a major reason for existence. Surely, reproduction is the key to species survival. The male seed (scientifically known as sperm or germ plasm) is produced by special cells, called Sertoli cells, which are neatly packaged in the many feet of tiny tubules that make up the bulk of the male sex glands, the gonads (testes), which lie in the sac known as the scrotum. Between these tubules (called seminiferous tubules) lie the interstitial cells (Leydig cells) which

Figure 11-1: MALE REPRODUCTIVE SYSTEM

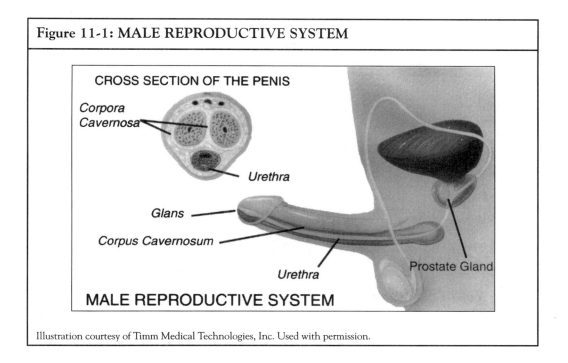

Illustration courtesy of Timm Medical Technologies, Inc. Used with permission.

are responsible for the manufacture and secretion into the bloodstream of the male sex hormone, testosterone. Both the seed-making and hormone-making functions are stimulated and controlled by the hypothalamic-pituitary gland's hormone secretions known as gonadotropins (LH and FSH). The scrotum hangs beneath the base of the penis and the testes are suspended thusly by the spermatic cord. The cord itself is a complex structure containing muscle (the cremaster), a reservoir (the epidydimus), blood vessels (spermatic arteries and veins), and the sperm duct (vas deferens). Despite the proximity to the penis, the sperm ducts must travel a tortuous route to reach the goal. Each duct (the vas) must travel through a canal in the groin (the inguinal canal) to dive into the main body cavity (peritoneum), where it terminates in the prostate and seminal vesicles (another storage facility). Semen itself, the liquid portion of ejaculation, is not made in the testes, but rather in the prostate gland. Sperm cells (spermatozoans) must climb a circuitous route using their inherent swimming, whipping tails, to be stored in the seminal vesicles and prostate, ready for action when called upon. Production of spermatozoa, interestingly, must take place at a

Figure 11-2: MALE URINARY SYSTEM

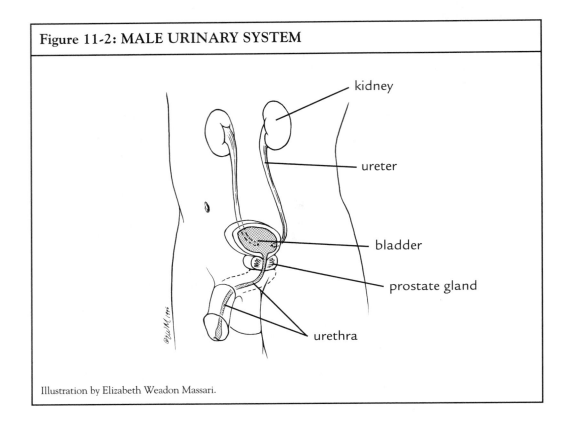

Illustration by Elizabeth Weadon Massari.

temperature of approximately 4 to 5 degrees F below body temperature. Presumably this is why the scrotum is where it is. You have noted, I'm sure, that your testicles hang lower in hot weather and conversely are hugged close in during cold exposure (the penis retreats a bit too in cold). This up-and-down bobbing is called the cremaster reflex. You may elicit it yourself by scratching the inside of your thigh with a well-pared fingernail.

Last, but by no means least, is the penis, an acrobat of great ability. It is one of man's most precious possessions and deserves the respect and care usually given to royalty. Penises come in all sizes, shapes, and colors and (similar to breast size in women) arouse great emotional anguish if they do not meet the usually unreasonable standards set by the media-influenced and susceptible ego. The medical advice in such cases is to relax. It's okay. Really. We'll discuss it some more later. Anatomically, this organ is composed of three closely bound, rodlike structures ending in a helmet-shaped knob known as the glans penis. The penile urethra is enclosed in the lowermost rod, while the two spongy erectile structures known as the corpora cavernosa lie on each side and on top of the urethral structure.

The cavernosa are capable of expanding and filling with blood when an ingenious set of valves at the venous outflow areas close. This retention and congestion of blood causes erection and widening and lengthening of the penis. This prevents urine flow but permits ejaculation when accompanied by the orgasmic, rhythmic contraction of the muscles of the external bladder sphincter and the prostate. After ejaculation (or even without it if sexual excitation diminishes), the vein valves open and detumescence occurs. If, for some reason, the valves do not open and erection is maintained abnormally, the disorder known as priapism occurs. This is named after a Greek god known as Priapus who was blessed and cursed with a constant erection. This is actually, in us mortals, a painful disorder requiring emergency treatment by a urologist. (Be careful what you wish for, lest it be granted.)

Common Genitourinary Disorders

Kidney

The large variety of disorders of the kidney would take volumes to discuss and can merely be mentioned briefly here. Nephritis, or inflammatory kidney disorder, is usually due to infection or autoimmune processes which may be initiated elsewhere in the body. True kidney infections (or pyelonephritis) may also occur. These usually originate from below due to obstruction and backflow from the prostate, bladder, or urethra. This is less common in the male than in the female. Here men are more fortunate; women are frequently afflicted by bladder infections due to the short female urethra and resulting easier bacterial access. Kidney infections may also be blood borne from infections elsewhere in the body. Urinary tract infections are serious matters and require prompt antibiotic therapy. People with this condition are usually quite ill, with high fever and pain in the flank or abdomen. Diagnosis by a physician is necessary for appropriate treatment to be instituted. Occasionally, pyelonephritis may be caused by the presence of a stone in the kidney. The crystallization of a variety of salts in the collecting portion of the kidney causes kidney stones. The chemical salts that are likely to do this are usually calcium salts (especially oxalates), which are highly insoluble in urine. Other substances, such as uric acid and cysteine (an amino acid) may also solidify and form a stone. Stone formation, therefore, frequently is a consequence of some metabolic abnormality of the body, such as an overactive parathyroid gland (calcium stone) or gout (uric acid stone). Stone formation, with or without metabolic disease, is frequently associated with dehydration. This causes the urine to become relatively thick and syrupy and will help crystals to form salts that accrete like stalactites in a cave. It is extremely important, therefore, that people who have had urinary stones (kidney, ureter, bladder) of any kind forever maintain an adequate water intake, especially in hot weather. Other preventive measures depend upon whether a metabolic cause can be detected. Excellent preventive measures are available in these cases. Treatment of stones, once they have formed, depends upon the location, size, and type. Small kidney stones (¼ inch or smaller) usually will pass through the ureter and into the bladder and out without major intervention. Such passage causes intense pain known as renal or ureteral colic, and has been likened to the pain of childbirth. Characteristically it starts in the back on one side or another and radiates, in a severe cramping style, down toward the pubic area of the abdomen. There is also frequently sympathetic abdominal cramping and nausea. Blood may appear in the urine, but even if not visible to the eye it may be seen via microscopic examination. In past times, larger stones which did not pass required surgical manipulation, either through special instruments inserted through the penis and up into the bladder or ureter, or occasionally, even open surgery to remove the most stubborn ones. Now, thankfully, most stones are readily removed by ultrasound pulverization (lithotripsy) from the outside of the body, an important milestone in urology.

Kidney tumors are generally bad news. They are usually malignant and may be "silent" until inoperable. Frequently they are diagnosed during a urologic evaluation for something else, such as prostate disease. Two points need emphasis. First, blood detected in the urine may be the earliest sign. This test is done as part of a routine urinalysis which in turn is part of a general checkup; another reason for these periodic tune-ups. Second, since many of man's ills are caused by smoking, it shouldn't shock you to hear that kidney and bladder tumors, too, belong on this dreary list of potential consequences.

Urinary Frequency

The volume of urine excreted during a twenty-four-hour period is determined by precise mechanisms. The hydration of the body tissues and the fluidity of the blood cannot vary too much without serious consequences. The hypothalamic hormone, vasopressin, is secreted in response to water deficiency or early dehydration. This hormone acts to decrease water excretion by the kidney and provides a thicker, more concentrated, darker yellow urine. Excess water turns off this mechanism and water flows freely through the kidney, up to 6 or more quarts per day, depending upon intake. The adult average urine volume for twenty-four hours is approximately 1 to 2 quarts. Over 2 quarts per day is considered potentially abnormal and is known as polyuria. This may be entirely due to excessive water drinking in people who do this, but this situation is not usual. It would keep one chained to the urinal, so to speak, and is a bother that most of us will avoid. In the absence of abnormal fluid intake, polyuria may signal disease. The most common polyuric disease is diabetes mellitus, or "sugar diabetes." The kidney is forced to excrete excess blood sugar, that which exceeds normal amounts. The upper level of blood sugar is about 180 mg per 100 ml of blood. Sugar greater than this amount is excreted into the urine with enough water to keep it dissolved. This is why diabetics are thirsty and drink excessively, and at the same time they are constantly running to the toilet. Sugar in the urine is easily detected chemically. The urine actually is sweet; hence the word *mellitus* meaning sweetness. In the days before chemical tests, the diagnosis was made by tasting the urine. The doctor's lot was not an easy one!

Certain hypothalamic and pituitary diseases, which are manifested by absence of the hormone vasopressin, also cause polyuria without sugar. This disorder is known as diabetes insipidus, with very insipid, colorless, not sweet, watery urine, up to 12 quarts per day. This relatively rare disease is now easily managed by the use of vasopressin nasal spray or injection.

Polyuria may also be produced by the use of certain chemicals which act on the kidney to produce more urine, the diuretics. (Despite the sound of the word, it has nothing to do with diarrhea.) There are a large variety of diuretics; some are natural, such as the caffeine in coffee or tea and some herbal types. But the most potent diuretics are drugs such as furosemide (Lasix®) or hydrochlorthiazide (Hydrodiuril®) which cause the kidney to excrete salt and drag water along with it. These medicines are very valuable in the treatment of diseases manifested by salt and water retention, such as congestive heart failure or liver cirrhosis. These diseases are associated with swelling of the extremities and fluid in the body cavities. Use of diuretics in such instances may cause rapid urination of many quarts (and pounds) of excess water and salt in a short period of time, to the great relief of the patient.

The number of times one must urinate daily depends not only upon the total daily volume of urine produced, but also upon the bladder capacity and other factors including, in men, the state of the prostate gland. Before leaving the kidney, it should be noted that urine production also depends upon the blood flow to the kidney; the more blood filtered, the more urine produced. Kidney blood flow will vary through the day depending upon gravity. More urine is produced when the body is horizontal rather than vertical. Gravity increases the flow to the kidney when one is lying down. More urine is, therefore, produced at night than when one is up and around during the day. Getting out of bed to pee during the night is not abnormal, but sometimes needs to be done urgently in the morning when one awakes.

Ureters

Not much trouble occurs here unless they are struggling to move a stone through (see page 178). Otherwise, these tubes usually conduct themselves benignly during our lives.

Bladder

The bladder, being a hollow, muscular balloon, has a finite capacity, usually about 1 quart without overstretching. This capacity varies depending upon a number of factors. First, thickening of the muscular wall will, paradoxically, decrease the capacity because excess muscle tissue takes up room. This situation most commonly occurs in older men because, with aging, the prostate enlarges and may cause some resistance to urine outflow. The bladder muscle responds to this just as any other muscle responds to harder work. It enlarges and grows stronger to meet the challenge. At the same time, bladder capacity falls and we older guys have to use the urinal more frequently, day and night.

Another factor affecting bladder capacity is irritability. Every muscle of the body has a certain irritable threshold above which involuntary contraction will take place. The most common cause of bladder irritability and inflammation in men is infection, usually arising from the prostate or the urethra. Inflammation of the bladder is called cystitis. Other types of infections, such as tuberculosis, are rare these days. Bladder irritability is manifested by frequency of urination, urgency ("I gotta go, *now*"), and occasionally incontinence. Nervous spasm of the bladder may occur in anyone during extreme fright or stress.

Stones may form in the bladder just as they do in the kidney, and when present are a cause of irritability, infection, and urinary frequency. Bladder stones, for some reason (perhaps dietary or hygienic), are far less common than they were a hundred years ago. One of the first surgical procedures done, beginning in medieval days, was "cutting for the stone." Since no anesthesia was available, the poor victim had to be held down by four strong men while the primitive urologist rapidly and neatly made an incision into the bladder from the space beneath the scrotum. Swiftly (in a matter of seconds) the bladder stones were removed. If the patient was lucky, he was stone drunk, so to speak.

Finally, a doctor needs to promptly evaluate and treat bladder polyps and tumors. The usual cause of these lesions (*lesion* is the medical term denoting any type of tissue abnormality, from a wound to a tumor) is thought to be chronic inflammation from chemicals or infections. This may be from exposure to industrial chemicals or dyes, tobacco usage, or (usually in the tropics) chronic parasitic cystitis. In this country, smoking seems to be the major culprit. Diagnosis is usually made by the discovery of blood in the urine on routine urinalysis. The bladder can be easily visualized through the penis using a narrow, lighted tube known as a cystoscope. Unlike the old days of being cut for the stone, the patient is properly anesthetized. The doctor can easily see and biopsy suspicious areas of the bladder. Polyps and tumors may be removed via this route. Total removal of the bladder is rarely necessary these days because of improvements in methods of treatment. Even if it is necessary, the bladder may be replaced using a spare loop of neighboring bowel to manufacture a new one.

Prostate

This important gland is discussed on pages 187–193.

Urethra

This tube, extending from the bladder through the penis to the outside of the body, may become infected, often through sexual transmission. There is one great convenience this tube gives us men. Think of it next time you are hiking; if your bladder calls, your exposure is comfortably limited.

Testes (Testicles)

These two oval bodies signify strength and determination in song and story. The term testament, both old and new, is a true derivation, by George. Giving "testimony," literally derives from the ancient practice of demonstrating ones testicles ("two of good weight") as a token of good, true faith and legitimacy. Things have changed, for sure, and such posturing is not only out of fashion but is usually detested and considered to be illegal and a danger to society.

The testes manufacture both seed (sperm) and the steroid hormone testosterone, upon directed stimulation of the pituitary gonadotropin hormones FSH (follicle stimulating hormone) and LH (lutenizing hormone), respectively. Testosterone, which is produced in large amounts only after puberty, is the male anabolic (tissue-building) hormone and is responsible for muscle and bone strengthening, beard growth, and all other virilizing features, including sexual desire and functioning. Here we will talk about some of the medical problems that may affect the testes and scrotum.

I have already mentioned the importance of checking one's own scrotum during the shower, the most convenient time. The shower is usually warm and the testes are well down from the body. One should be able to feel the entire globule on each side. Sometimes there is only one. It is unlikely that this will be a new discovery to most adult males, since usual childhood examinations detect the absence of one or both testes in the scrotum. This condition, known as undescended testicle or cryptorchidism, arises when the primitive gonad (testicle) remains in its prebirth embryonic position inside the abdomen. Cryptorchidism, if detected in infancy, requires surgery to bring the gland down through the inguinal canal into the scrotum, where it is secured. A cryptorchid testicle is still able to make testosterone, but it cannot make sperm because of the higher body temperature. One-sided cryptorchidism in the adult is most common. One testicle is all that is needed for fertility. The major concern in adult cryptorchid men, is the higher incidence of testicular cancer developing in the abdominal testicle. Prior to the development of sophisticated imaging machines like the CAT and MRI scanners, exploratory surgery was frequently recommended to detect and remove the internal testicle. Now, a negative CAT scan or MRI showing no evidence of problems usually suffices to avoid surgical exploration.

Examination of the scrotum and testicles is of the utmost importance to detect abnormal lumps or nodules, which could represent testicular cancer. These tumors used to be most dreadful and incurable, but happily now they are almost always curable with appropriate surgery and chemotherapy, particularly if detected early.

Occasionally inguinal hernias, the most common type in men, are felt as lumps in the groin or scrotum. These are usually painless and will disappear when one lies down and the hernia contents go back into the abdominal cavity unless they are incarcerated or stuck. Hernias are very common and are not dangerous unless they become strangulated (these are usually very painful and swollen and are surgical emergencies). These days hernias are fixed with in-and-out surgical repair. These are so-called "Band-Aid" surgeries, with fortifying mesh left in to strengthen and repair the weakened bulging groin area. Disability is usually only a few days.

Penis

Penile infections and discharges will be discussed later in a separate section dealing with sexual diseases. Several other items need mention here.

Circumcision. This has become quite a controversial subject in the past few decades. This surgical removal of the foreskin (or prepuce, the sleeve of skin that slides over and covers the tip of the penis) is a fairly routine procedure in many hospitals in the United States. The procedure has been suggested for all boys for hygienic reasons, although the American Academy of Pediatrics has recently come out with the dictum that circumcision is no longer recommended. The circumcised penis is easier to keep clean. Circumcision prevents infections, known as phimosis, with painful adhesions of the penile glans (tip). Another concern is that of prevention of cancer of the cervix in the partner of the individual. This tumor is rarely seen in the mates of circumcised males. It is not certain, however, that this is still the case, since the sexually transmitted disease herpes type II and human papilloma viruses (HPV—genital warts) may be important factors, and circumcision does not prevent these. Penile cancer and some sexually transmitted disorders seem to be prevented and are, at least, less common in the circumcised. (Penile cancer is rare in any case.) Finally, some experts believe that AIDS and other sexually transmitted diseases are less easily passed to and from the circumcised penis. This is suggested by statistics from African and Asian countries where heterosexual AIDS in the male is frequent, unlike in the United States where circumcision is common.

These data and suggestions notwithstanding, the opposition to circumcision as a routine practice (except in the case of religious requirement) has gathered passionate support in recent years. Such slogans as "the rape of the penis" and "ritual child abuse" have been used by the "Antis," who point out that this anachronistic procedure is cruel, painful, and devoid of scientific proof of efficacy. The effect upon sexual functioning and enjoyment of such is debatable. Philip Roth, in one of his novels, quotes his heroine as preferring the uncircumcised organ for "playing with" and the "bobbed job" for intercourse and oral sex. Male patients have begged me for circumcision to increase enjoyment, while others regret the absence of the foreskin for the same reason. My own feelings are less intense than either position. Certainly if one's religious faith requires this procedure, there is no argument. I personally do not feel, however, that the operation, in this day and age, can be justified by the fear of future medical disaster. I do think that if circumcision is done, even to newborns, adequate anesthesia is a necessity.

To summarize, circumcision has its potential advantages, but seems to be entirely elective, unless one has strong feelings, religious or otherwise.

"Bent Penis." This is a peculiar and mysterious condition which usually affects men in mid- and later life. The medical name for this distressing problem is chordee or Peyronie's disease. For unknown reasons a plaque of scar tissue develops on the top portion of the penis, and by preventing full expansion during erection, bends the penis either moderately or, more often, mildly out of the straight. Actually, there is a normal tendency for the penis to have a slight bend when erect with a mild upward, banana-like concavity. In chordee situations, the bend may be severe enough to interfere with insertion into the vagina. Total interference is rare and obviously needs some treatment. If it is mild and intercourse is possible, even with some fancy manipulation, it is probably best left alone, because frequently the deformity will abate by itself. Treatment consists of surgical removal or incision of the plaque or injection of cortisone. These methods are only partly successful and sometimes not at all helpful, unless an internal splint is implanted; not an easy operation. Patience and understanding by the sex partner is preferable in these cases.

Priapism. This is a rare condition of involuntary, prolonged, or persistent painful erection. It may be caused by blood disorders such as sickle cell disease (most common in the black population), where the penis outflow valves may be blocked by a blood clot, keeping the cavernous rods of the penis distended with blood. Certain medicines (some antidepressants such as trazadone) or chemicals (papavarine) also (rarely) cause this problem. The hormone prostaglandin E may, if injected, produce erection of some persistence, which actually may be useful in certain cases of impotency. Priapism needs prompt urologic attention for relief.

Fertility

Something strange is happening in the world. The fertility of almost all male animal species, especially Homo sapiens, seems to be declining at a rapid rate. For reasons that can only be surmised at this time, the quantity and quality of semen and spermatozoa have been decreasing throughout the world. It is of little consolation that the insect world is doing fine, fertilitywise. Biologists are speculating wildly about this phenomenon. Theories have been proposed, some of which seem quite reasonable. For instance:

1. Lifestyle, especially use of drugs (particularly marijuana), alcohol, and cigarettes, plus increased stress, may be major factors. These unwholesome habits have been scientifically known to decrease sperm quality and number.

2. Pollution, toxic chemicals in the air we breathe and the food and water we eat and drink, may have similar deleterious effects on sperm production.

3. Pesticides may be a factor. Of particular concern are some pesticides (DDT, chlordane, and so on) which apparently have some hormonal activity blocking reproductive processes. DDT, for instance, decimated some bird populations by interfering with eggshell formation. Human tissues also are capable of absorbing and storing these substances and experts worry about the effect they will have on human sexual functioning.

4. Estrogens (female hormones) are known to adversely affect the prenatal male. This was determined when the effect of DES (diethylstilbesterol) on the babies of pregnant women was ascertained, years after the practice of giving this artificial estrogen was abandoned. (It was given during the forties, fifties, and sixties to prevent miscarriage.) Genital anomalies including cryptorchidism, deformities of the penis, and low sperm count were seen in some of the approximately one million sons of these women. (The daughters developed other problems, notably vaginal tumors of a rare type at an early age.) While DES is no longer used, the presence of estrogens in food (meat from animals given hormones to increase growth) is under suspicion. Even more worrisome is the suspicion that many industrial chemicals may masquerade as estrogens by binding to our hormone cellular receptors. These chemicals, such as dioxin and PCBs, are found everywhere, but especially in highly developed industrial environs.

It is almost as though nature is trying to tell us something about our human frailty and the consequences of our exploding population and its dependence upon technology. The sperm count of our grandfathers (in the range of 120 million per milliliter) was almost twice the average male count today in most developed countries where such studies have been done. Despite this, the incidence of male infertility, while yet small, is of concern. If the trend continues, and particularly if nothing is done to reverse it, we may, as a species, be facing a bleak future. In the meanwhile, the fact remains that it takes only one healthy sperm to make a baby and even with low counts (below 20 million/ml is considered the infertile range) medical science has developed ways of concentrating spermatozoa. It is even now possible to inject a selected healthy sperm into an ovum via *in vitro* (test-tube) fertilization techniques.

What can be done to prevent infertility? Little, it would appear, aside from avoidance of suspect chemicals and drugs, tobacco, marijuana, and excess alcohol. The tight-underwear theory (overwarming the testicles decreases sperm production) is widely promulgated, but is probably overstated. Some urologists perform removal of varicose veins of the scrotum in an attempt to cool the testes, but this operation has not shown great results, to my knowledge.

My advice here is to cool off, not the testicles, but the attitude. Infertility need not be diagnosed until at least six to twelve months of trying. Incidentally, spontaneous pregnancy in infertile couples who have adopted in frustration is by no means rare. It suggests again a powerful neuroendocrine effect on human reproduction. Fertility workups are complex and expensive and should not be hastily done, in my opinion.

Prostate

A book that deals with men's health will, of necessity, have a separate section dealing with the prostate. This is an exocrine gland that is strategically placed surrounding the neck of the bladder. It functions to produce semen liquid and also acts as a sperm reservoir which empties with ejaculation. Prostatic fluid itself is a complex mixture of sugars, enzymes, and other substances which sustain and help motivate the sperm toward its goal. It is a mischievous organ. Its own function and size is dependent upon the male hormone testosterone and its hormone derivative (after enzyme action on testosterone), dihydrotestosterone. This chemical conversion, as you shall see, is important. In the absence of dihydrotestosterone the prostate cannot grow and function properly. It may actually shrink. If the prostate gland enlarges, as it does in the majority of men with time and constant hormonal stimulation, it may cause narrowing and pressure on the urethra as it leaves the bladder. This is a normal and frequently distressing outcome of aging in the male. It is known as benign prostatic hypertrophy (BPH). The degree of obstruction to urine flow is variable. About 75 percent of men over the age of sixty-five have some degree of BPH. About half of them are bothered by it. The bladder muscle compensates by getting stronger and thicker, making urination possible, though often more frequent. If the bladder is permitted to overstretch, as it may during the night when urination is inconvenient and postponed by sleep or laziness, urination may be difficult and prolonged in the morning. The same difficulty may be noted in other situations such as cold weather, excessive alcohol use, and use of bladder muscle–weakening drugs such as antihistamines, decongestants, codeine-type painkillers, and some antidepressants. The absolute worst scenario is that of acute urine retention, which occasionally occurs, often in conjunction with one of these precipitating factors. In such cases, catheterization of the bladder to remove the urine and permit the bladder to regain its strength is necessary. One can usually prevent this painful event by being aware of the process of bladder emptying. The great Napoleonic Marshal Ney is said to have warned his army to "Keep your powder dry and your bladder empty, mes amis." Good advice to this day. The treatment of benign prostatic hypertrophy has changed in recent years and continues to change, with new options rapidly appearing.

First, it should be stated that treatment is necessary only if symptoms warrant; that is, if a man is willing and able to tolerate the inconvenience of urinary frequency and the need to get up during the night to urinate. No harm is done by doing nothing else, so long as urinary retention is not great and infection and kidney damage due to back pressure is not present. Avoid the aggravating factors; needlessly "holding it in" and taking drugs and medicines which are known to weaken the bladder.

Recent advances in pharmacology provide major help with symptomatic BPH. The prostate gland contains involuntary muscle cells which, when relaxed, loosen the grip of the gland on the urethra. New drugs, the so-called alpha-blocking antihypertensives (Hytrin®, Cardura®) are effective in relaxing these muscle cells and relieving some of the obstruction. These medicines have proven very effective in about 50 percent of cases. Another drug called finasteride (Proscar) has been developed to ingeniously block the conversion of testosterone to dihydrotestosterone, which is the prostatic-active hormone. This medicine has been available for a few years now and it appears to be effective in about 50 to 60 percent of cases after use for six to twelve months. (You will recall that the same drug, sold in half-strength size tablets, is marketed as an antibaldness remedy under the name Propecia.) The prostate gland actually shrinks to some degree. Also, this same drug is being used today for an anti–prostate cancer effect (not yet proven, but promising). The drug must be taken continuously (one pill per day) and is generally well tolerated. The major side effects reported by some patients include diminution in volume of semen during ejaculation and, in a small percentage of men, some loss of sexual desire (libido). It appears now that a majority of men who suffer from prostatic symptoms may be treated with these medicines (one or both, if necessary) successfully, particularly if they are willing to put up with some urinary frequency and night rising.

Recently the herbal remedy saw palmetto has been used to treat BPH symptoms. A recent review in the *Journal of the American Medical Association* reported that it "may" help to ease the symptoms and "seems" to have fewer side effects than finasteride. As with all the others, this natural substance has not been thoroughly tested but seems to be harmless. As with all the other naturals I must withhold my recommendation, at least for the present.

The alternative to medical treatment is surgical manipulation of the prostate by a variety of methods. The "gold standard," a term used by urologists for this procedure, is transurethral prostatic resection (TURP). This procedure removes much of the obstructing prostatic tissue through the penis, utilizing a cystoscope with an electric cutting wire loop. The prostate gland is located and carefully chipped away by this means until obstruction is relieved. Recovery time in the hospital is generally about three to four days or until catheters can be removed and the patient is able to urinate freely on his own. This is not a minor procedure to be sure, and bleeding and discomfort are regular postopera-tive events to a greater or lesser extent, but these problems are manageable. Many patients are ecstatic at the results. "Freedom at last," claimed one patient to me a few weeks after his TURP. "Now I can put a campfire out again. It's like playing with a new water gun." Others have not been quite so happy. For one thing, retrograde ejaculation, that is, backflow into the bladder rather than ex-ternally, is the norm after this surgery. Also, for unknown reasons, a number of patients complain of decreased sexual desire and potency, although there is no known reason for this. (Urologists tend to discount this, but I'm convinced that it happens.)

Removal of the prostate by open surgical means, usually through an ab-dominal incision, is actually safer than TURP, according to urologists. Bleeding is more easily controlled and the prostate can be simply shelled out of its capsule like an orange from its peel. The prostate is more completely removed and recur-rence of prostate symptoms, which can happen with TURP, is unheard of. The late side effects are the same as for TURP, but hospitalization may be a bit longer. This procedure is particularly appropriate for those who have huge prostate glands which cannot be adequately removed through the penis.

There are some new techniques that may offer a substitute for these more radical ones. Laser-beam prostatic surgery through the penis is supposedly less bloody and better tolerated than conventional TURP, but the evidence is not yet in. Recently approved by the FDA is a nonsurgical technique which seems quite promising. This is placement of an electrodiathermy catheter into the prostate portion of the urethra through the penis and heating the prostate gland (via this shortwave energy) for an hour or so. Allegedly this causes more or less perma-nent shrinkage and relief of obstruction with no cutting at all.

Prostatitis

The prostate gland, having connections via the urethra inward (to the bladder) and to the outside, is subject, in this strategic location, to infection from above or below. Direct infection from the adjacent rectum has also been implicated but probably doesn't happen unless contamination is introduced directly, such as by a biopsy needle. In any case, the highly susceptible gland (semen is a very desirable growth medium for bacteria) is subject to infection, both acute and chronic (smoldering). Infection is manifested by the usual pain, tenderness, fever, and swelling characteristic of such events, and the victim may be quite ill. The diagnosis usually is not too difficult to make because of the symptoms of urinary discomfort and frequency and the occasional presence of pus, blood, or urine which appears unusual. Sometimes, however, the diagnosis is not clear. Rectal examination and prostatic massage should always be done in cases of unexplained fever in a man. The material that is massaged out of the urethra and onto a slide usually shows characteristic pus, which may then be cultured to determine the type of germ and its antibiotic sensitivity. Treatment with appropriate antibiotics is quite effective. The length of treatment depends upon the type of infection. Hot baths are helpful (it may be easier to urinate while in the tub). Occasionally, with chronic infection, repeat massages may be necessary until the infection clears. Incidentally, prostatitis has been blamed on too much or too little sexual activity, but there is no proof either way.

Prostate Cancer

This is probably the most vexing subject in male medicine. It is filled with ironies and paradoxes, conflicting facts and figures, fears and failures. Fact: Prostate cancer is the third most frequent cause of male cancer death in the United States (in 1995, the number-one cause was lung cancer with 158,000 deaths, number two was colon-rectum cancer with 46,000 deaths, and number three was prostate cancer with 41,000 deaths). In 1996, new prostate cancer cases will exceed both of the other two combined, according to the American Cancer Society. The irony is that with the current screening techniques available, more early cases are being detected. The paradox is that most of these cases will probably not cause the death of the victim. It is estimated that if a man lives to the age of ninety, a prostate cancer will be found if looked for at autopsy more often than not. The fear is that if the early detected cancer is left alone without radical intervention, it will kill its host, even though we know now that probably a majority of these cancers will not progress to clinical disease (the bearer of the tumor will probably die with it and not from it). Our failure is the fact that at present we have no adequate way to determine which cancer will behave aggressively. We can only guess, based on certain variables such as age, severity at the time of diagnosis, tissue appearance under the microscope, certain chemical tests (PSA), and the general health of the patient. Also, despite improvements in therapy, we cannot guarantee cure in all cases even if the indications suggest otherwise. Despite all, it is generally accepted that prostate cancer screening is an important and major advance in preventive medicine. This consists of finger examination of the prostate via the rectum, combined with a new blood test, the prostatic specific antigen, or PSA. This test measures a substance that is manufactured solely by prostatic tissue and is released into the bloodstream. The PSA blood level is determined by both the size and activity of the gland and its cells. A large prostate, therefore, such as in BPH, will generally have a high blood level as will, at least theoretically, a cancerous one with its actively enlarging cell numbers and size. Unfortunately, as yet, we cannot tell the difference between benign or malignant PSA. Therefore, digital (finger) prostate examination must be done at the same time as the PSA test. In a questionable situation, elevated PSA with a bumpy or otherwise suspicious-feeling gland, the next step will be an ultrasound examination of the prostate. This is easily done, without pain, through the rectum. If the doctor detects any questionable areas by this technique, a rapid needle biopsy, guided by the ultrasound picture, can be done readily. It is a relatively easy and painless procedure and it has made definitive cancer diagnosis a simpler matter, though one cannot be sure from the biopsy what the prognosis of the cancer will be. The patient and his doctor will then be faced with some difficult choices.

What are the alternatives? If the cancer appears to be in its earliest stages, confined to the prostate gland itself (various tests including MRI of the area can be done to ascertain this), radical prostatectomy can be performed. This surgery, which removes the entire gland and its capsule (and frequently lymph nodes in the area), is curative in about 75 to 90 percent of the cases. Sadly, impotence, despite the much touted nerve-sparing procedure developed by Dr. Walsh of Johns Hopkins, is a frequent and expectable outcome of this surgery. Also, incontinence to some degree is common. Despite this, and also the dangers of any surgery, most men, in my experience, opt for this chance for enhanced survival, although as I've indicated, it cannot be guaranteed. Indeed, statistics cannot demonstrate any difference in survival years in untreated men with low-grade cancer versus the general population. The trouble is, again, we cannot truly distinguish the aggressive from the nonaggressive types even where, in many cases, the cancer is limited to the prostate alone.

Other treatments offered for this disease include radiation therapy, which seems to be highly effective in many cases and doesn't cause incontinence, although it does cause impotency fairly frequently. Hormonal treatment, consisting of male hormone removal (by castration) or suppression by taking drugs, has been used as an effective anticancer therapy, though efficacy is usually limited to a few years.

The dilemma is apparent. My advice to patients is dependent upon their needs but it would appear logical to me that men under the age of sixty-five have the greatest reason to opt for the aggressive surgery, while those over age sixty-five (centainly over age seventy) apparently live just as long without it. Each case must be judged on its own merits and the patient's informed wishes. It is hoped that refinements in the PSA test (differences in PSA produced by benign versus malignant cells) will someday tell us more about the prognosis of this disease in its early stages. Researchers are looking for such noninvasive methods to give us this vital information.

DR. DASHE'S TIPS FOR HEALTH MAINTENANCE

1. Self-examination of the scrotum and testicles is as important to a man's health as breast self-examination is important to a woman's. Make it a point to examine yourself once a month for lumps or anything else out of the ordinary.

2. If you live long enough you will have some type of problem with your prostate. The dreaded rectal examination is a vital part of early detection of problems, make sure it is a part of your regular examination.

3. You have a 50 percent chance of being the source of any fertility problems. If you and your partner are trying to have a child without success, you should be the first one to be tested; sperm counts are easy to do and less invasive than testing for a woman's infertility.

4. The decision on circumcision has already been made for you at this point. If you have a son, you and your spouse will be the ones making the decision. Religious reasons notwithstanding, the controversy rages on about the hygienic and aesthetic reasons for circumcision. This won't be the last tough decision you'll have to make as a parent.

5. Hernias and other ruptures in the groin canals are very common and easily repaired with improved surgical methods.

6. Urinary tract stones are painful. The most frequent cause is dehydration so keep your water intake up, especially in hot weather.

7. Detection of prostate cancer has become easier via the PSA blood test, ultrasound, and needle biopsy. Choice of treatment can be difficult, but cure is more likely with early detection.

Chapter 12

MALE SEXUALITY AND SEXUAL HEALTH

The good news is that despite the derailment of the sexual revolution by AIDS and other sexually transmitted diseases, healthy sex is still alive, well, and as delightful as ever. The bad news is that this is a truly terrible development that will forever change our thinking, practice, and our lives.

The revolution started with the work of Alfred Kinsey (*The Kinsey Report*, 1947) in the mid–twentieth century. Kinsey, an insect morphologist, decided to study, by scientific statistical means, the actual sexual practice of American men, something that had never been systematically done before. Sure there were oodles of marriage guidebooks available, usually tucked away in one's parents' night tables. Sneaky kids could steal a glimpse when the cat was away and get the same misinformation that mom and dad had. The main source of sexual lore for boys of my generation was the street. Street talk was probably no more misleading than the sex manuals of the day. Kinsey pointed out that what people actually did was highly different from what was purported. For starters, he found that almost all men were sexually active, one way or another, for most of their lives.

Just about everyone masturbated without evident harm. About 20 to 30 percent of men admitted to some form of homosexual practice sometime during their lives (usually boyhood or early teens) when, in those days at least, heterosexual activity was relatively rare for young people. Dr. Kinsey, in a 1952 lecture that he presented at the University of California Medical School, made the point that in his judgment our species was "omnisexual"; that is, depending upon the culture and the circumstance, people will practice one form of sex or another, even if it is limited to shaking hands with your dog. This view seems a mite extreme, but there clearly is some truth to it (for example, the high incidence of homosexual activity in prisons, single-sex boarding schools, and cultures where homosexuality is not frowned upon, such as in ancient Greece).

In any case, Kinsey started something; much research and investigation, via confidential survey (the *Hite Report* and many others) and even laboratory observation (Masters and Johnson) have followed. For better or for worse, our laws and attitudes have loosened and relaxed—I think perhaps in some ways to an extreme. The overuse of sexual profanity and posturing in everyday life, especially in the media has, in my opinion, robbed our society of something, subtlety and gentility at the least (and I am no prude). Honesty and openness are beneficial though, and all in all, our enhanced knowledge has been for the better. We need to know more about ourselves and denial of the truth has been harmful. Even pornography, whether one finds it distasteful or not, has not been shown to incite perversion. In studies of this issue (especially in Scandinavia), the incidence of sexual misconduct is markedly diminished by the availability of pornography. We need to educate our children and ourselves to protect us from harm, internal and external; such is the beginning of healthy sex.

Sexual Preferences

This is a touchy subject. Opinions vary from the fiery, Bible-thumping right to the angry, overpermissive left, and the reasonable approach is usually crushed between the two. One does not have to be a religious fundamentalist or the Marquis de Sade to argue vociferously on the matter; even the scientists do. It was not until about ten years ago that the official Psychiatric Classification of Disease removed homosexuality from its listings. The presence of the considerable population of openly practicing homosexuals has made this status more or less acceptable to the law, if not to much of the general population. Acceptance is slowly being achieved now, and barring a swing to the fundamentalist right, may soon gain full legal acceptance. There are probably still many "closet" homosexuals, those who can hardly be blamed for hiding because of the stigmatization that still is present in our not-too-gentle society.

Some scientists are convinced that there is a genetic basis for homosexuality, which many homosexuals claim, too. They feel it is not simply a preference, but a necessity. To them, there is no choice. There is some evidence for this (some anatomical features suggest feminine characteristics in the brain structure of male homosexuals). I believe that this evidence is not yet convincing enough to most scientists, and even though I may be labeled politically incorrect, I tend to agree with Kinsey's theory of omnisexuality.

Sexual Practices

I have previously expressed some disdain for how-to books dealing with sex, but there are now a few exceptions. One of them, *Male Sexuality* by Bernie Zilbergeld, is particularly valuable for what I have called bibliotherapy for the individual who needs detailed information on the subject. I recommend Zilbergeld's book for deeper exploration than what I can provide in this book.

Masturbation

First, let us deal with solo sexual practice, which is truly safe sex with obvious advantages. Not only is disease avoided, but so are charges of sexual harassment and the legal and social hazards of dealing with a sexual partner in these litigious times. That is, if one avoids the more kinky and adventurous methods of masturbation utilizing vacuum cleaners, whips, chains, nooses, and such infernal devices. Masturbatory methods have perhaps been fancified by devices made available via mail order, advertised in *Playboy* and its clones, but basically it still consists of manual stimulation of the penis while active mental fantasy is exercised. Let it be said again and again, masturbation is harmless and even beneficial. It cannot cause hairy palms, blindness, or any other curses. It may relieve stress and tension. Frequency of the practice is also unimportant, and it is socially harmless if done privately.

Sex with Others

The sexual revolution really revved up in the 1960s with the discovery of "the pill" by Gregory Pincus and others and the subsequent freedom from fear of pregnancy by many women. The apparent conquest by antibiotics of serious venereal disease relieved other fears. No longer was virginity a virtue to much of our youth. There seemed to be no reason for restraint in the sixties and seventies. Recreational drug use abetted disinhibition. The Kennedy assassination, Vietnam, and Watergate seemed to effect a general cynicism and demoralization which has, sadly, continued to this day. Commitment to old moral standards, and for that matter to anyone but oneself, seems pointless to many. Divorce rates have rocketed. Young people marry, if at all, later in life than before and single-parent families are now commonplace.

In the late 1970s the state of California, realizing that medical schools were seemingly deficient in the teaching of human sexuality, mandated that a postgraduate course in human sexuality be necessary for continued medical licensure. My wife and I attended the first certified course in human sexuality, presented by the University of California, in 1978. Attendance by couples was strongly encouraged. It was interesting. The material, at first mildly titillating, soon became mind numbing and rather boring. Still, the law is the law. My medical colleagues and I dutifully finished the course and went back to our practices loaded with information that had been previously considered salacious and taboo. I fully expected that patients, singly or in couples, would now be calling upon me to act as a sex teacher-guide. To my surprise, I found that my patient population seemed to have few such questions. The level of technical sophistication was high. Books, movies, and TV had already spread the word. Marital and interpersonal problems were not due, I found, to lack of technique but almost always to communication problems. It dawned on me that people who will not or cannot talk to one another cannot have a close relationship, sexual or otherwise. Herein lies most of the sex difficulties. During the sixties and seventies, promiscuity and casual sexual activity was the norm; closer relationships were not apparently needed or desirable, as in the past.

Then came herpes, then genital warts, and finally AIDS—the great monster that ate up the revolution. People were and are, if they bother to consider the consequences, scared of casual sex. Unfortunately, too many people, especially younger ones, are not so careful. The baby boomers have outgrown their wild days and have taken up monogamy and marriage. Many younger people, though worried, still apparently take chances with unprotected sex. I shall discuss AIDS and the other sexually transmitted diseases later, but this is my main point regarding sex with others: not only is casual sex perilous, it is not nearly so fulfilling and pleasurable as a true connection between lovers. Married or not, great sex requires emotional commitment; whether you call it love or something else.

So if it's technique you're after, let me refer again to the easily available and quite explicit sex manuals, particularly *The Joy of Sex* series by Sir Alex Comfort. Incidentally, I am awestruck by the incredible lead and cover stories now featured in the used-to-be pious ladies' magazines, *Glamour, Redbook, Good Housekeeping*, and so on. Don't those ladies think of anything else? Times have surely changed.

Sexual Practices with Others, Including "Safe Sex"

I'm not going to tell you how to "do it." You probably know. There are a few things, however, that should be emphasized. First, assuming the absence of transmissible disease and the desire of one's sexual partner, there are few sexual practices that are physically harmful. Of course, if there are religious or other deeply felt inhibitions, these must be considered and those practices avoided. Ask before you do it. Oral sex, mutual masturbation, licking, sucking, massaging, touching, kissing are OK; go ahead, as long as you are confident with whomever you are sharing bodily fluids. One practice that is not so safe or comfortable, however, is anal intercourse. For one thing, it may be painful and repulsive to the recipient. For another, the anus and rectum are not designed for such use and though the act may be pleasurable for some, there are potential problems, even other than AIDS; for instance, inflammation of the rectal tissues, spread of intestinal bacteria to the genitalia, and flare-up of hemorrhoids. Anal intercourse, if done at all, should always be done with a condom (removed immediately afterward and, of course, discarded) and plenty of soap and water (penis and anus). This goes for both sexes. Clearly, if performed, it should be done slowly and gently (never mind what the latest porn films show. Porno stars have plenty of medical trouble, believe me.) The rectal membrane cells are particularly receptive to the AIDS virus. This is the reason for the rapid spread of this plague through the Western world's homosexual population. Female rectal cells are also not protected, and it has been found that many of the early cases of AIDS in women were detected in those women who engaged regularly in anal intercourse, usually with multiple partners. Heterosexually transmitted AIDS was, until recently, relatively uncommon in the absence of this practice.

Bodily fluids and responsible sexuality. Bodily fluids are saliva, semen, mucus secretions from any orifice, urine, breast milk, liquid feces, and blood. All of these may have some capability of carrying and transmitting disease organisms to another place or person. Responsible sexuality should include avoidance of such disease transmission. The only certain way of doing this is to abstain from sexual contact of all kinds. Blood transfusions, though best avoided if possible, are now reasonably safe with the new testing methods. Contact with contamined needles, such as occurs with drug addicts, is almost certain suicide. Tourists to AIDS areas in Africa and Asia are advised to take their own disposable syringes and needles in case the necessity for injection arises.

   Bodily fluids differ in their capacity to transmit infectious agents. The organisms themselves are choosy. For instance, gonorrhea germs may be present in vaginal, penile, and also rectal secretions, but the disease is not known to be transmissible by sweat, blood, or urine. Sweat, incidentally, is the least likely to carry any disease germs, so it's quite safe to shake hands with people. We will, in a later section, deal with each of the sexually transmitted diseases in more detail, particularly hazards and modes of transmission. At this point I wish to make some most important general statements.

Healthy sex is not only safe sex but sex with fulfillment and joy, release and comfort. This not only is hygienic but aesthetic. The safe part is easier. Limit your sexual partners to those whose safety concerns are as great as yours. Take *no* chances with decisions made at a time of passion. At the very least, use a *latex condom*. Be as sure of your partner as you are of yourself. If necessary, be tested and insist your lover do the same.

The aesthetic part is a far more complex business. Sexual healthiness may be defined in many ways, depending upon your own standards of morality, religion, and sexual preference. After hearing and seeing the dramas and the outcomes of the many human relationships, happy and sad, laid on my physician's desk, I am no longer willing or able to easily judge what is healthy. There are many ways of love, and life and times are dynamic and ever changing. There seems to be no absolutes, except perhaps that experiencing love and sex is a marvelous gift of life, not to be feared or shunned. Feeling nothing, being alone, is hell.

Premature ejaculation and impotency. These are subjects worthy of some discussion, despite my previous resolution to avoid "how-to" lecturettes. Premature ejaculation refers to the unfortunate, anxiety-related occurrence of orgasm with semen emission, either prior to or too soon after vaginal penetration. It is almost always a problem of the young and inexperienced man, usually with a similarly inexperienced (and to make things worse, usually frustrated) partner. Biologically speaking, rapid ejaculation is all that nature calls for. In almost all cases, this problem is caused by what is rightfully called performance anxiety; again, it is almost always in a young, potent, impatient man whose excitement takes over. A well-choreographed act of intercourse requires adequate time for foreplay and then, after intromission, sufficient time for enjoyment by all. This is a fine concept but it is very difficult to accomplish when someone, namely yourself, is watching and timing the action. This self-observation can and does frequently lead to either rapid ejaculation (sometimes even before insertion) or, even more humiliating, loss of erection and ruination of the whole episode. The scenario that follows next depends, of course, upon the actors. Such phrases as, "Don't worry baby, it could happen to anyone" (sweet and kind), or "Dammit, what the hell's wrong with you?" (mean and vile) are of little help. Before I mention the possible preventive management of this sad situation, a few reassuring facts are in order. First, the very fact that ejaculation occurs at all should be celebrated. It essentially rules out any serious physical sexual problem. One has to have an intact nervous system, blood supply, and glandular function to reach this point. The second fact to remember is that orgasm is not automatically granted to every act of intercourse. It is estimated that the average is 70 percent for men and 30 percent for women. Several things can be done. First, talk to your lover about it. It can be a great help to simply understand the problem. Second, welcome the first rapid ejaculation simply as a prelude for the second bout of intercourse as soon as your refractory period (time before you are able to do it again) is over. The second time usually takes longer. Third, try the "squeeze" technique. This is where the partner takes the glans penis between thumb and index finger and squeezes moderately firmly. This usually stops ejaculation before it becomes inevitable. Zilbergeld's and Comfort's sex books will cover this in greater detail. In any case, once a man gets a bit of confidence and experience, the problem usually goes away and stays away. Recently, certain of the newer Prozac®-type antidepressants (SSRIs) have been used in the treatment of this condition. These drugs have a frequent side effect of delaying orgasm and, therefore, may prevent premature ejaculation effectively.

Premature ejaculation is considered by the sexologists to be a mild form of impotency, and I suppose technically it is. If so, it is the easiest form to treat and cure. The other kind, inability to achieve or maintain an erection or ejaculation, is not a simple matter. Rather, it is complex and a subject of much writing and research. It is also a common and serious medical and psychosocial problem, despite the many jokes associated with it.

Unlike premature ejaculation, true impotency may be caused by a failure of one or more links in a complex chain. It is the job of the physician to detect and treat the defect; that is, if it cannot be self-treated adequately by getting and using accurate information. (Bibliotherapy, again; Zilbergeld's book can be very helpful here.)

The first and probably most common form of impotency is the so-called psychological or primary type. Our old nemesis, performance anxiety, is the principal culprit but other simple psychologic factors may play a major part. For example, incompatibility of the lovers can cause problems. Sexual dysfunction may be the language used by partners to consciously or unconsciously communicate dissatisfaction with a relationship. This, rather than lack of technical know-how, is the most common cause of marital sexual failure and the reason for the proliferation of the many marriage and family counseling services we see nowadays. I have referred such patients to appropriate therapists (some are better than others) with mixed results, I fear. Modern life seems to strain partnerships, particularly long-term ones.

Any psychological disturbance may result in impotency. Depression, for instance, is a frequent underlying factor. Unfortunately, treatment for depression, using the latest antidepressant medicines, may also cause the same sexual problem. Indeed, medications of various kinds have been shown to have deleterious effects on sexual functioning. These include, in addition to antidepressants and sedatives, anti–high blood pressure drugs, diuretics and even antihistamines. Endocrine disorders involving the sex glands, pituitary gland, or the hypothalamic part of the brain which controls the pituitary function can manifest impotency as the presenting and major symptom.

As an endocrinologist, I have had occasion to see many patients referred to me for impotency. But endocrine evaluation is only part of the diagnostic process. A disorder with so many potential causes, even multiple causes in the same individual, is a tough diagnostic challenge to a physician. Such examination must be done before treatment, which is usually very effective, can be instituted.

Before undergoing a major search for a physical cause of impotency, a rather simple device may be tried to distinguish psychological from organic types. This depends upon the phenomenon of nocturnal erections, which may be associated with dreaming and REM (rapid eye movement) sleep. Nocturnal and morning erections are indications of intact physiology, hormonal, neurological, and vascular. This sleep-time activity may be measured (at some expense) by use of a penile pressure measuring device and recorder (a pressure strain gauge, sometimes called a penometer). More simple, and a lot cheaper, is the use of a roll of perforated postage stamps. The appropriate length is glued around the base of the organ at bedtime. A torn stamp perforation in the morning indicates erection during the night. These and other screening diagnostic maneuvers may be helpful but persistent impotence requires a full diagnostic workup.

First, the physician must do a thorough history and physical examination. Intercurrent and previously undetected diseases, such as early diabetes, may be at the root of the problem. Other illnesses take precedence over reproduction in our bodies when it comes to utilization of resources. Obviously, a thorough genital examination must be performed to check the basic equipment. Neurologic examination is important to detect nervous system disease which can interfere with the erectile mechanism. Erection requires intact nerve connections from the spinal cord to the penis. Vascular examination is necessary to detect possible obstructed or impaired blood flow to the penis; this is usually due to arteriosclerosis. Blood tests, including the routine ones previously mentioned, are important. For example, blood sugar studies are necessary to rule out diabetes, a very common underlying cause of impotency.

It is now possible to measure the blood levels of the sex hormones, particularly of testosterone and the pituitary gonadotropins (the hormones that stimulate the testicle to make testosterone). If the testosterone level is less than normal, the stimulatory hormone level should be elevated. If both levels are low, it may mean a brain or pituitary deficiency, which could result from a tumor or other disease of this area. A particular pituitary hormone called prolactin which has no known specific function in the male (it is necessary for lactation in nursing mothers) is measured. If the blood level is high, it may signal the presence of a pituitary tumor known as a prolactinoma. This particular type of tumor, which makes an abnormal amount of prolactin, will cause severe impotency. Fortunately and happily, the disease is reversible and the tumor treatable without surgery with the use of an antihormone medicine known as bromocriptine. These particular hormone tests, therefore, are vital in medical testing for impotency.

These endocrine diseases are far more common than previously thought, and current hormone therapy is useful. I have been impressed in recent years by the finding of an abnormally low blood testosterone level, associated with a normal pituitary gonadotropin level but no x-ray or other evidence of pituitary or brain disease. My suspicion, without proof, is that something in our environment, chemical or psychosocial is causing this. I have the feeling that much research will be necessary to ferret this out. In the meanwhile, treatment consisting of testosterone administration may be effective. This male hormone is best administered in the form of long-acting injections (Depotestosterone® [testosterone cypionate]) taken every two to four weeks. Oral male hormone tablets are available but are potentially harmful to the liver, since oral medication must first pass through this organ, and large "hits" seem to cause damage. Testosterone skin patches have been recently developed, but they are relatively expensive and must be used daily to maintain adequate blood levels. Incidentally, testosterone administration is important for treatment of all manifestations of testosterone deficiency, not only for restoration of potency. Because this substance is the anabolic (tissue-building) hormone of the male, deficiency can lead to bone and muscle loss, anemia, and other problems.

Further treatment for impotency relies, of course, upon the cause, which is frequently undetectable even after thorough examination. In our medical frustration, we tend to call this primary, functional, or psychological impotence. Whatever the cause, treatment is necessary and available.

Psychologic treatment, usually involving intensive counseling, may occasionally use a sex-surrogate therapist. The surrogate is a highly paid expert who will take an impotency victim, by mild and gentle stages, through the process of sexual intercourse. Shady as it sounds, some experts recommend it, although there are no statistics available regarding success. Less wild, perhaps, but at least occasionally effective, is the counselor's advice for the patient to avoid anxiety by the simple means of having a nonpressuring sexual experience. This means doing everything except trying intercourse, for a period of time. The expectation is that eventually intercourse without anxiety will happen. Whether this works or not, it's worth trying. Too frequently, though, this and all the other counseling stratagems do not seem to help much. Many physicians, myself included, will then suggest moving on to the next empiric step. Whether or not it's scientific, if it works, everyone is happy. Testosterone administration seems to help some people, even though blood levels may be normal. The reason for this may be that there is an active form of the hormone that is biologically more important than the rest, which may be chemically bound to blood proteins and rendered inactive. Whatever, some of my colleagues will hate me for saying this but a shot or two of testosterone is worth trying. Testosterone is a known libido (sexual desire) stimulator, in women and in castrated men. I believe it may do the same in normal men if their blood testosterone levels are on the low-normal side; certainly if they are even just a little below the line. (I have no way of proving this, I admit, but I think it's worth trying anyway.) There is some evidence now that additional androgen in the form of testosterone given in small doses may actually help prevent some of the physiologic and psychologic decline of aging, loss of libido and potency included. Many experts in the field of impotency management express the same opinion. Everyone who has a potency problem has, as a result, a psychologic potency problem from then on. It is unhelpful to stand stodgily on scientific principle and not offer assistance in the form of more active measures. It will help the psychological block in any case, if confidence in one's ability to achieve erection can be restored. Other measures are as follows:

1. *Medications.* Prior to 1998, there were few consistently effective potency restorers. Testosterone, as discussed above, worked sometimes in appropriate cases and, of course, bromocriptine in the case of prolactinoma. There are a few instances of drug side effects (i.e., priapism or libido stimulation) with such medicines as the antidepressants trazidone and Serzone® and the anti-Parkinson's drug L-dopa. These could not be used for their inconsistent potency effects, and they have potentially far more onerous side effects. Yohimbine, an old natural remedy derived from the bark of an African tree, affects the sympathetic nervous system to stimulate potency and libido in a few patients (perhaps 10 to 20 percent), and since it was inexpensive and relatively safe, it was not infrequently tried. From time immemorial, herbal nostrums, remedies, and homeopathic drugs from ginseng to rhinoceros horn have been touted by entrepreneurs in various cultures, including our own, as aphrodisiacs (libido and potency stimulators).

   Then—hallelujah—came Viagra (sidenafil), a drug that was originally investigated as a blood vessel expander. It works by causing an enzymatic-chemical release of nitric oxide into the tissues, in this case the penile corpora. Nitric oxide, it appears, relaxes the smooth muscle of the penile blood vessels, permitting engorgement and erection of that organ, but only, miracle of miracles, if there is sexual stimulation. Ergo, it does not cause unwanted erection or priapism, but in a majority of cases it will produce enough of an erection to permit satisfactory intercourse. It appears to work even in situations that appeared to be unlikely, such as post-radical prostatectomy, severe diabetic nerve disease, and even in vascular insufficiency. It is not 100 percent effective, incidentally, but in doses of 25 to 100 mg it works in a majority of cases. There are few side effects for most men; these being transient visual disturbances, headache, flushing, and dyspepsia. There have been a number of cardiac deaths reported in men who have used the drug, but it is generally believed that these have occurred in men with previous severe cardiac risk factors, some of whom may have precipitated heart crises by being too exuberantly sexually active. Precautions, therefore, have been issued in such cases, and the drug is contraindicated completely in those men who use or require nitroglycerine in any form for heart disease.

The bad news is that Viagra is expensive (at the time of this writing, it costs from $8 to $12 per pill in pharmacies in California). Insurance plans may or may not cover the cost, unhappily, and much angry politicking is being carried on as I write. Incidentally, it has not been shown that Viagra may be a sexual aid in women, but theoretically could be, and there is much discussion and even prescriptions written for this purpose by some gynecologists.

To summarize, Viagra works for impotency much of the time but not always. It is not an aphrodisiac, and emotional causes of impotency may not be helped. It is my understanding, by the way, that the FDA frowns upon the scientific search for a true aphrodisiac. But, the way things are going in national politics . . . ? In any case, Viagra has opened the door to more effective and tolerable anti-impotency drugs, and more are on the way. Just watch the newspapers. Before leaving the subject, one tragicomic digression may enlighten and amuse. It is well known in pharmacology that poisons of the strychnine type cause a pre-lethal discharge of the autonomic nervous system associated with erection and orgasm. The Japanese blowfish, otherwise known as fugu, is known to have a deadly strychnine-like poison in its liver. The flesh of the fish is delicate and much enjoyed eaten raw as sashimi, usually by very wealthy men. If the special chef (they are intensively trained and licensed) serves a fugu dinner and, by error, it has been said, contaminates the sashimi with the liver poison, the diners may die and the chef is then duty-bound to commit suicide. This story, when I first heard it seemed unbelievable and then, after some thought, seemed an example of the Japanese love of the aestheticism of danger. Subsequently, I learned from an article on the subject in the *Scientific American*, that the true story is slightly different but no less romantic. The chef is supposed to make a tiny slit in the liver, letting just enough of the poison into the sashimi to cause a mild, non-fatal poisoning, manifested by general excitement, tingling, erection, and possibly orgasm. That's what I call a fancy dinner!

2. *Vacuum devices.* Suppose Viagra doesn't work? For years *Penthouse*, and other sex magazines have been hawking various penis-enlarging devices consisting of a hollow plastic tube into which the penis is inserted. A hand vacuum pump at the other end is worked to supposedly enlarge the organ. It does much of the time, temporarily. The vacuum causes negative pressure to pull blood into the penile corpora cavernosa, distending them and causing erection. If a rubber band is immediately placed around the base of the penis, erection may be maintained long enough for vaginal penetration and successful intercourse. This technique was borrowed from the porno advertisers and is now legitimately manufactured and sold as a (expensive, of course) useful medical device. (The price is about $300 to $500; about ten times more than the sex toy.) This requires some training and practice and a supportive partner is essential for success, but it works and many physicians and clinics are prescribing it. It is especially useful for impotency due to diabetes and nerve or blood vessel–type impotency.

3. *Penile injection.* There are chemical substances that, when applied directly into the penile tissues, will cause prompt and sustained erec-

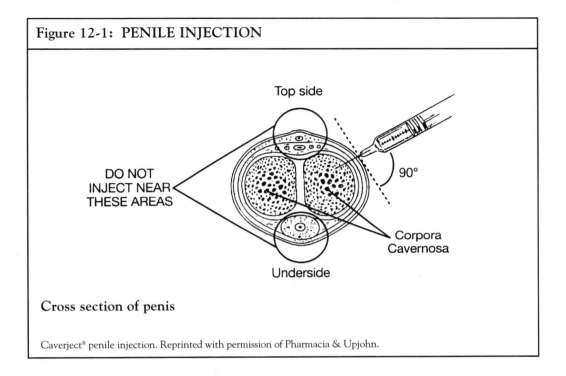

Figure 12-1: PENILE INJECTION

Top side

DO NOT
INJECT NEAR
THESE AREAS

90°

Corpora
Cavernosa

Underside

Cross section of penis

Caverject® penile injection. Reprinted with permission of Pharmacia & Upjohn.

tion. Unfortunately the only way is to inject the stuff directly into the corpora cavernosa. This was the subject of the medical lecture of the century, given by a famous urologist to his colleagues at a major urologic meeting. The good doctor, after describing the process, dropped his pants, showed his flaccid organ, turned around, injected his penis, rotated again and demonstrated to the awe-struck audience a magnificent erection. Thunderous applause followed. The substances used include papaverine (an alkaloid derived from opium but with no narcotic action), Regitine®, and alprostatel (a prostaglandin hormone). Used separately or together in minute amounts, it is injected with a fine hairlike needle into the penile base (Figure 12-1).

In most cases, whatever the cause of impotency, a competent erection will happen and intercourse may be performed. As horrifying as it may sound, injecting one's own penis at the base is not difficult nor painful once learned in the doctor's office. It is quite a safe procedure with only rare and controllable side effects (prolonged erection). That first step, however, getting over the idea, is a big one. The FDA has just released, for patient use, one of the injectables (Caverject®). Research continues in this area. It is possible, for instance, that substances rubbed into the penis or inserted into the urethra may gain enough absorption through the skin to do the trick. One such substance under investigation is nitric oxide, which is a natural blood vessel dilator. All of these intrapenile drugs apparently work by aiding venous valve closure while increasing arterial flow into the penis, thus generating an erection even without intact nerve input. Another similar technique available worth mentioning is called MUSE®. This works by insertion of a pill directly into the urethra with a skinny applicator. This too is an unpleasant technique and thought to most men, but it does work in the majority of cases, though not quite so effectively as injection.

4. *Penile implants or splints*. Professor of urology Robert Pearman, now deceased, was a friend, colleague, and sometime patient of mine. About thirty-five years ago I attended a lecture of his dealing with organic impotency. We in the audience noted that Dr. Pearman used as a blackboard pointer a rather long (2 foot) bone that was unrecognizable to us. He reviewed the field as it existed at that time, and then came to his dramatic purpose. His pointer was the os penis of a walrus. An os penis is a bone of the penis (os = bone in Latin), and many animals, including walruses, whales, and many rodents, are blessed with these penis stiffeners. Dr. Pearman is generally credited with the discovery of the human penile implant. Pearman performed many implant procedures early on and now it is an accepted method of devising a permanent erection capable of vaginal penetration. It is, of course, a major and expensive surgery but it works, and many men have been happy with the results. I must warn, however, that this surgery be done by a highly skilled surgeon who is very experienced in the operation. I have seen tragic failures when done by the wrong hands. There are a number of variations of the implants, all of which are of two basic types; one permanently stiff, and a more inge-

Figure 12-2: PENILE IMPLANT

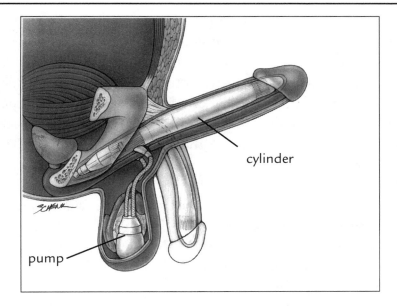

AMS penile prosthesis. Courtesy of American Medical Systems, Inc., Minnetonka, Minnesota.
Medical illustration by Michael Schenk.

nious prosthesis that may be flaccid and when desired, manually pumped up for the desired erection (the pump is in the scrotum—the pumper can be either partner, see Figure 12-2). This clever device is far more expensive and more prone to later mechanical difficulties than the permanent penile splint.

Finally, before leaving the subject, it is of vital importance that patients realize that vaginal intercourse is not the be-all and end-all of healthy sex. There are many ways of making love, and many couples enjoy sexual fulfillment and pleasure with the closeness and deep feeling achievable with massaging, touching, kissing, or oral contact; bringing one's lover to ecstasy may be, in the last analysis, the healthiest and happiest part of human sex.

Penile Lengthening and Enlargement

In the past few years, beguiling ads have appeared in the media (usually on the sports page) claiming miraculous procedures that lengthen and widen the male organ, all for only a few (five to ten) thousand dollars. When I first saw these ads, I guessed that the charlatans were on to a new thing. Nothing had, as yet, appeared in the medical literature that could explain how such procedures could be possible. The following information was obtained from some respectable urologic colleagues. There is a penile lengthening procedure, of sorts. The surgery consists of the cutting of some of the ligaments that hold the penis to the pubic bone of the pelvis, thus permitting the base of the penis to drop down about an inch. There is no true lengthening of penile tissue. The circumference and width of the penile shaft is augmented, albeit temporarily (for weeks or months) by the injection of fat cells under the penile skin. The donor sites are usually from the buttock or abdomen. I cringe at the thought of this mutilation and I wonder at the desperation of those who seek it out. This is my opinion, although I admit I have not seen the results of this surgery. I understand that one of the original surgeons has had some legal problems about this procedure. However, the ads are still there. Caveat emptor.

Male Contraception

Women don't trust us much when it comes to responsibility for birth control. I don't blame them. Not only is our gender more prone to mindless hormone-driven passion, it takes only one wriggly seed to do the trick. I have seen sufficient instances of "pregnant virgin" syndrome (where ejaculation occurred without penetration), that I have come to believe it really exists. I strongly urge women to take the final responsibility for contraception. Of course, one must not forget that an unwanted pregnancy caused by the erroneously confident male is no laughing matter. So, everyone should be involved. I shall not deal with female modes of contraception here, but it's a good thing for a sexually active male to find out about them. There are only a few ways for a man to have reasonable certainty about his own contribution. These are condoms and vasectomy.

Condoms. The proper and constant use of a latex condom is paramount. Condoms come in all shapes, sizes, colors, and designs with external textures and "ticklers" if one is so inclined. There are two principal types, however, and this is important: Latex condoms, made by major, reliable companies (check with *Consumer Reports* if you're not sure) are safest, both for contraception and even more important, to prevent passage of sexually transmitted disease organisms, particularly AIDS. In addition, the kind that contain the spermicide nonoxynol-9 are better for this purpose. The other types, mainly sheep membrane or synthetics, are not reliable for disease blockage. The condom must be placed properly on the penis before *any* intromission and must be held on firmly upon withdrawal and discarded immediately. One should then wash the genitalia with soap and warm water before further sexual activity is initiated. Some couples even make a pleasant, sexy game of the process.

A word about potential male contraceptive drugs: They are being developed, but they all have some serious drawbacks that make them unreliable or troublesome. They are still experimental. For instance, paradoxically, the administration of large doses of male hormone (including steroids such as the ones some athletes use or abuse) will suppress and even eliminate sperm production. This, however, is not entirely reliable for contraception. It is important, though, for the users to be aware of the likelihood of infertility.

Vasectomy. This procedure, consisting of tying off or removing a segment of the sperm tube (the vas deferens is the anatomic name, hence vasectomy) interrupts the flow of spermatozoa from the testes to the prostate and seminal vesicle storage facilities. The vas is a long tube, extending from the scrotum, through the inguinal (groin) canal, into the abdominal cavity where it meets its terminus at the prostate-bladder junction. The surgery is simple, since the part of the tube that is worked on is in the scrotum and the surgeon can easily feel it. The procedure is generally done in the urologist's office and takes only a few minutes. The vasa are held and brought up to the skin of the scrotum, a tiny incision is made on each side of the scrotum, and the tube exposed, cut, and tied firmly. The two ends are clearly identified and both are placed back and the incision sewn. Easy, unless there is a third vas hiding someplace. It does happen, though rarely. This is why a semen analysis must be done in about a month or so to make sure that the surgery has worked and all sperm emission halted. It almost always does. To be certain, the patient should not have unprotected intercourse until this final analysis is completed; residual sperm may remain in the prostate for a while. Semen volume will not be altered. Vasectomy is safe and probably the only certain method of male contraception, barring castration (removal of the testes) itself. It has never been proven to have deleterious effects on the body, despite some unestablished claims that have been made. A few patients have complained of decreased libido and potency afterward, but there is no proof that this is a result of the surgery. More likely it happens, I suspect, if the patient is brought into surgery by his wife (holding his ear), saying to the urologist, "Here, I want him fixed!" Incidentally, it is possible to reverse the procedure years later (the sooner the better for a successful result). Although the testes cease sperm formation when the tube is tied, the sperm-producing Sertoli cells may be able to regenerate and begin production, if the procedure is reversed.

Sexually Transmitted Disease

I well remember the military movies that demonstrated the ulcerated, gangrenous penises that resulted from thoughtless dipping into the "vaginas from hell" that surrounded our nice, clean, military facilities. Those were simpler and happier times, in regard to venereal disease. "Short-arm" inspections were carried out weekly in barracks, and gonorrhea and syphilis victims ferreted out for treatment and punishment. Gonorrhea, caused by the bacterium gonococcus, and syphilis, caused by a spirochete (spiral bacteria) called treponema, were the common venereal diseases of the day. They still exist and can cause big trouble but they have taken a backseat to the new sexual plagues. This is because gonorrhea and syphilis are still sensitive to antibiotics and relatively easy to cure. It is truly a sad irony that the sexual revolution which seemed to liberate us so has given us so much pain and travail as the price. Somehow it seems unfair but not unexpected; there is still no such thing as a free lunch.

Gonorrhea (Clap)

This old-timer causes, primarily, urethritis (inflammation of the urethra) with painful urethral pus discharge on urination. If left untreated, it can involve the scrotum, the joints, the bloodstream, and even, rarely, the heart. The doctor can easily diagnose it by bacterial examination of the penile discharge and it is easily treated by antibiotics. Although the gonococcus germ has gradually become resistant to certain ones like sulfa and penicillin, we still have drugs that work. The first symptom is usually pain on urination with greenish discharge from the penis. Ptompt treatment is essential. Condoms prevent it.

Syphilis

This historically fascinating illness is thought to have been brought to Europe by Columbus's crew from the New World in the 1490s. At least, it did not seem to appear until then. At the time, it was almost as savage and deadly as AIDS to that nonresistant and unimmune population. Over the years it has become a far less violent disease with the population seemingly less susceptible. However, it is still a serious and potentially fatal illness if not treated. It has three stages, the first manifested in three to six weeks after sexual contact (with genital secretions) by a painless ulceration of the genitalia known as a chancre. This heals rapidly without treatment and all remains quiet for two to six months until secondary syphilis occurs, manifested usually by some form of rash and fever. If this remains untreated, tertiary syphilis may develop in about a year. This may be a truly devastating disease which can involve the brain and spinal cord, the heart, blood vessels, and just about every other organ in the body. The spirochete may lay dormant without apparent disease manifestations. This is known as latent syphilis. Blood tests will detect it, as well as the active forms of syphilis. The spirochete itself may be seen by microscope if the original chancre's secretion is examined this way. Though it certainly exists and even may be increasing in frequency, as are many infectious diseases, syphilis is comparatively uncommon. Perhaps this is because the microorganism is still sensitive to penicillin, one of our first and best antibiotics, as well as many of the others. Antibiotics are used so often now for good (and bad) reasons, it is possible that syphilis has become suppressed as an unintended but fortunate result.

Chlamydia

Chlamydia trachomatis is a nasty microbe that causes, in men, nongonococcal urethritis (discharge and burning) as well as, less often, diseases of the scrotum, urinary tract, rectum, and lymph nodes. This vicious bug causes trachoma, as its name indicates, a major cause of third world blindness from eye infection. Recently it has even been suggested to be involved in causing coronary artery disease by infecting susceptible arteries. We'll see. What next? Lymphogranuloma venereum, once thought to be a separate viral venereal disease, is now known to be caused by chlamydia. It is treatable with antibiotics and usually responds well. The diagnosis is frequently made by exclusion (if gonorrhea germs are not found), and curative treatment with doxycyline and other antibiotics is usually commenced. This organism is particularly malicious for women, since it can cause deep pelvic infection and subsequent sterility. It is terrible also for the newborn, causing severe eye and lung infections. Condoms prevent sexual transmission.

Genital Herpes Simplex (herpes simplex type II)

The only positive thing that can ever be said about AIDS is that it has taken the heat off herpes type II. It is sad to recall the fear and anguish expressed by the young patients whose painful genital blisters destroyed their own personal sexual freedom. Even now, it remains a cause of inordinate remorse and loathing that is really not justified, for it is not a new disease. It is a member of the chickenpox, fever blister group of viruses, and it has always been with us. It is almost identical to the oral fever blister, type I herpes, and, for the male at least, holds no great danger, though it may be uncomfortable and recurrent. Like the oral type, herpes

II never totally disappears, although it usually remains asymptomatic and latent unless stirred up by excess heat, friction, or other inciting factors. It is more of a problem for women in whom, it has been theorized, it is a possible precursor for cervical cancer. Even more insidious is herpes at the time of childbirth. A newborn who contracts herpes II in the birth canal is in great danger of developing congenital herpes, which can be fatal. Pregnant women are now regularly tested for herpes at the time of delivery. Fortunately, herpes type II is treatable with the antiviral agents acyclovir and famcyclovir, which lessen the duration of pain and viral shedding, and may also, if taken regularly, prevent recurrence. It is rarely necessary to take medication on a regular, ongoing basis for the disease; fortunately, it is usually only sporadic. Condoms prevent transmission and should be used by any male who has had herpes and any man who has sex with a woman who has had herpes lesions (active or not). Should herpes prevent a long-term relationship? My opinion is "No." If people love each other, they can live with herpes. They must simply be aware of the potential problems and act accordingly. In addition, herpes may lie dormant for years, and the sudden appearance of this disease does not mean recent infection; i.e., a deception by a sexual partner. The disease may have been lying in wait, as it were, for years. Also, it should be realized that type I herpes (oral) may be transferred to the genitals via oral contact.

Genital Warts

Another serious problem, especially for women. This, too, is not a new disease; it is more widespread and apparent because of the revolution, with its increase in incidence of multiple sex partners. Genital warts are caused by human papilloma virus, usually type 6 or 11. Some other types (16 and 18 particularly) may be associated with precancerous changes of the female cervix or anus. Warts are otherwise not dangerous, but are unsightly and bothersome. There is no way of eradicating them except by various methods of direct destructive removal, such as the application of caustic chemicals such as podophyllin or liquid nitrogen by a physician. There are also self-administered topical medications available (by prescription only at this time). Genital warts tend to recur a lot and require retreatment and can be very annoying.

Chancroid

This is another rare oldie which is caused by a germ called *Hemophilus ducreyi* and is uncommon in the United States. Tourists to other lands need to watch out. It is treatable with antibiotics.

Pediculosis and Scabies

These are distressing infestations by insect parasites. Pediculosis means pubic lice infestation or "crabs" (also known as, amusingly, "seam squirrels" and "jock rabbits"). It is quite embarrassing but easily managed with topical lotions or shampoos (Kwell® or Nix®). Scabies (a mite) is also sexually transmissible and treatable (with Elimite®). Both partners and all laundry must be treated, for these parasites are easily transmitted.

AIDS

What more can be said about human immunodeficiency virus (HIV) disease that has not already been hammered at you by now? HIV almost always leads to AIDS (acquired immunodeficiency syndrome) and is now the leading cause of death among people twenty-five to forty-five years of age. The actual disease has an incubation period of up to ten years, indicating the time of contracting the virus was usually in the teens and twenties. Unhappily this pattern seems to be ongoing. Older sexually active people are more wary and careful. Another frightening thought is that experts now recognize that new strains of HIV are more easily spread by routine heterosexual contact. The kind we have previously seen usually required blood contact or anal intercourse for transmission. (These practices are more easily avoided.) One hopeful note is that we are now seeing a few patients who have apparently been spontaneously self-cured of HIV. At least, proven HIV-positive victims have become negative to testing. Also, some patients continue to have long-term HIV without apparent progression to AIDS. Perhaps the human species is becoming more resistant to this plague, just as happened in the history of mankind with other plagues such as syphilis and measles. Maybe we will find a cure or a vaccine that will eradicate the disease, as with smallpox. At least we now have better treatment, and much research is being done. The addition of the protease inhibitor type of drug to the previously available ones has, in many individuals, brought about remarkable remissions of AIDS, even in desperately ill patients. Occasionally, the virus can no longer be detected in the blood. Alas, it seems now that, despite this, the HIV remains hidden in cells in such patients, and return of the disease is being seen more often. Better treatment and prevention (e.g., an effective vaccine) is still necessary. We treasure these hopes and should never lose them, but we must face the facts of epidemiologic life. An overpopulated planet is bound to be at increasingly greater risk of unbridled new disease.

In the meanwhile, use your common sense and your latex condoms, preferably those that have nonoxynol-9 (my wife suggests decorating them with team logos or fancy designs).

DR. DASHE'S TIPS FOR HEALTH MAINTENANCE

1. It bears repeating again and again. Unprotected sex just isn't safe. Wear a latex condom if you can't be celibate or monogamous.

2. Impotence can be a result of either physical or emotional problems. Your doctor can isolate the problem, and new breakthroughs are occurring all the time in helping overcome the problem of impotency. Don't let your delicate ego keep you from taking advantage of new advances.

3. Masturbation is no longer considered a perversion and might have some health advantages.

4. There are a number of books, tapes, and devices created to enhance your sexual life. A good knowledge of technique and options will keep the spice in your sex life.

5. Despite your technical knowledge, the key to good sex is having a relationship that is built on understanding and emotional connection—more difficult to obtain but much more satisfying than good technique.

6. Penile lengthening and enhancement techniques are dangerous and should be shunned except for medically legitimate reasons.

7. Vasectomy is a safe and effective means of male contraception; other than condoms, it is the only one currently available.

8. Did I mention that unprotected sex is not safe?

Chapter 13

MENTAL HEALTH

A recent government survey estimated that more than fifty million Americans suffer from a mental or addictive disorder at any given time. I am somewhat dubious about such estimates because the definition of mental disease, which used to be a lot clearer, is now blurry and quite dependent upon the definer.

I would like to seriously try to define mental health and its disorders in some useful and meaningful way. It is impossible to come up with a simple answer. In my opinion, if one can manage to function in this difficult and trying world of ours, that individual is pretty healthy. Healthy, but not necessarily happy. Functioning in a dysfunctional world requires stamina, forbearance, patience, and not a little native equanimity. Driving to work, unless you are very lucky, has become a stressful, exhausting chore, and one is surrounded on the freeway by anxious, angry faces. By the end of the day, even if nothing untoward happens, you are a frazzled wreck. You may want a drink or two. You're tight as a drum. Are you mentally unwell? If you are so defined, then I think the government statistic missed about two hundred million other Americans.

Our minds and bodies have mechanisms that are able, for the most part, to deal with the slings and arrows of life. This is not a free ride. All of us, from time to time, suffer anxiety, depression, even physical illness when our defenses are breached or overtaxed. A man may wonder whether he is under special stress, work related or other. I believe that we are, indeed, subject to psychosocial pressures unique to our sex, so much so that I have devoted an entire chapter to this question because of its importance; it has to do with the requirements for healthy manhood in this incredible era of the millennium. While dealing specifically with mental health and disorders, a few points should be made regarding our sex.

1. We men are brought up to believe that we must stifle our emotions and tears, that there is something unmanly in reacting visibly to things that hurt and disturb us. Therefore, we tend to keep things within that need expression. This adds immeasurably to our mental distress.

2. Men deal with emotional turmoil differently than women. We tend to seek solace by running away to lick our wounds, or to seek comfort with alcohol or other self-destructive modes. Men are at greater risk of suicide than women. (It is statistically found that highly correlated variables in successful suicides are being male, white, middle-aged or older, alcoholic, single, and with a family history of suicide.)

3. We are frequently troubled and frustrated with our sexuality, since we are hormonally driven but forced by the rules of civilized society to curtail our feelings and actions. I would guess that most men have secret lives ranging from healthy, nondestructive fantasy (the great majority) to horrifying and aggressive acting out, for example, murder.

4. We are far more reluctant than are women to seek help for our emotional problems. Again, this is partly because of our obsession with strength and the need to conquer everything, including our own problems. Failure at this, which is almost inevitable, leads to greater anxiety and deeper depression. Frequently we will not seek help unless forced to by marital crisis and discord, pressure from friends or superiors, or a judge.

The most serious cases of nervous breakdown are marked by symptoms so severe that we cannot function in our jobs, our family lives or, in the maximum, life itself. Suicide may be the result of the extreme. Statistics show clearly that suicide rates are directly proportional to stresses at certain times of life (adolescence, menopause) as well as socioeconomic upheavals. I think that we are in the midst of one of these upheavals; hence the violence, fear, anger, and confusion that we read and hear about constantly, and that we may feel ourselves to some degree at some time. These intermittent feelings are entirely normal, so long as they do not interfere with our functioning. When they do, some form of assistance is needed. In any case, we all are in constant need of some help. Help comes in many forms, from friends, family, spiritual advisers, or significant others. It doesn't matter, as long as it works and it is not destructive. For instance, acting out in a violent fashion may help relieve one's rage level, but the consequences are dire. Drug and alcohol use may provide temporary solace and peace, but the cost can also be devastating. Let me be reassuring to this extent: you're OK if you are occasionally anxious or depressed. It is, ironically, healthy to be so if the circumstances warrant. I worry about the person who appears happy and cheerful at inappropriate times. I worry most about the person who feels nothing at all.

What Is Mental Illness?

Some definitions are necessary. The terms *neurosis* and *psychosis*, in use for about a hundred years, have for the most part been supplanted in the psychiatric community by more complex and supposedly more precise diagnostic terminology.

Neurosis

Simply stated, neurosis or psychoneurosis is defined as relatively mild personality disorders marked by excessive anxiety, depression, indecision, and some degree of social or interpersonal maladjustment.

Psychosis

Psychoses are more serious conditions characterized by impaired contact with reality. People with psychoses may frequently be plagued by delusions, paranoia, hallucinations, or withdrawal. These illnesses generally are now thought to be due to major brain biochemical disturbances. Researchers believe these distur-bances are usually brought about by genetic defects.

Character Disorders

Character disorders are manifested by socially undesirable behavior and lack of control of impulses without anxiety, guilt, or conscience. There is an inability to maintain relationships. Such individuals are frequently labeled psychopaths or sociopaths, depending upon how destructive is their behavior.

These are the major categories of mental illness. Prior to the end of the nineteenth century, such subtleties did not exist. Psychotic individuals were thought to be possessed by demons and were frequently ostracized or placed in asylums where they languished until death. Psychopaths were usually imprisoned or executed whenever they were caught, unless they were royalty or very rich. The advent of Jamesian and Freudian psychiatry changed that. Freud made the brilliant discovery of the unconscious and its relationship to human behavior. For a good part of this century, Freudian theory was the basis for much of psychi-atric diagnosis and treatment. Since the mid–twentieth century, major discover-ies in brain anatomy, physiology, and chemistry, along with the discovery of mood-altering drugs, have drastically changed the course of psychiatric history. There is no question that all of our behavior, intellect, and emotion is dependent upon our genetic makeup, our brain chemistry, and our environment. The influ-ence of each certainly varies with the individual, but all must be considered in the evaluation and treatment of mental disorder. This causes much controversy in the field of psychiatry. Economics has also intruded into the picture. The dis-covery of drugs that controlled the major manifestations of psychotic illness was the proximate cause of the decision to free the inmates of the mental asylums, supposedly saving much money for the taxpayer. Unfortunately many, if not the majority of these patients, now live on the streets and do not regularly take their necessary medications. Psychoactive drugs and psychotherapy by practitioners are also very expensive. Insurance companies and governmental agencies are al-ready dictating the type and duration of treatment of mental disorders. The future, I fear, bodes far more of this. I'll try to outline some practical stratagems for dealing with this problem. First, I'll define some specific disorders and problems more thoroughly.

Mental Disorders

Anxiety Disorders

Generalized anxiety refers to states of mood discomfort ranging from mild feelings of tension or apprehension to terror or panic. It is very much like fear without any obvious external threat. Typically, it is the feeling of "flight or fight." For example, if a bear is coming at you, such a response is well warranted. If you have the same feeling without the bear, that's clinical anxiety. This may be a temporary or a long-lasting state, but if it persists, it may be considered a manifestation of depression with anxiety. With anxiety, one may have actual physical symptoms such as sweating, racing pulse, rapid breathing, or hyperventilation. Frequently, people suffering from anxiety seek relief from drugs or alcohol.

Panic and phobia are varieties of anxiety. The person with panic disorder suffers from recurrent attacks of severe anxiety with signs and symptoms of fear and terror: sweating, trembling, palpitations, and an increase of depth and rate of breathing. The increase in breathing may lead to hyperventilation, which causes the blood to become too alkaline from excess loss of carbon dioxide. This alkalosis results in numbness and tingling, weakness, faintness, and spasm of the extremities. The individual, in the meanwhile, feels that he cannot fill his lungs sufficiently so he breathes harder still, making it all worse. Slowing the breathing and rebreathing into a paper bag brings almost instant relief of hyperventilation symptoms. Usually the afflicted person is not aware of any precipitating factor, but once begun he may associate the episode with the setting, producing at times a phobia such as agoraphobia (fear and avoidance of public places) or claustrophobia (fear and avoidance of enclosed places). There are many types of phobias that give rise to panic attacks. Compulsion and obsession, which are related to panic and anxiety, refer to uncontrollable urges to do things that may avoid anxiety episodes. For example, the obsession that disease-causing germs are everywhere, ready to attack, may cause an individual to compulsively wash his hands every few minutes. Obviously, these are serious and incapacitating problems which require professional help. There are, fortunately, medications and therapy available that often successfully control these situations.

Depression

The other very common mood malady is depression. This feeling of hopelessness, low self-attitude, and despair is also often masked by physical symptoms such as lack of energy, fatigue, loss of appetite for food or sex, weight loss, vague headache, stomach complaints, and so on. Bouts tend to recur and frequently there is a family history of depression. The problem ranges from mild blues to major psychotic episodes. When unreasonable euphoria (mania) alternates with depression, it is known as bipolar disorder or in the worst instances, manic-depressive psychosis. Brain scientists are convinced of a chemical basis for most depressive disease. One reason is that it is intimately associated with the endocrine epochs of one's life (adolescence, premenstrual syndrome in women, menopause, male midlife changes); another reason is the remarkable effects of the neurochemical antidepressive medicines.

Substance Abuse

Substance abuse refers to alcoholism and drug abuse. These are, in my opinion, related to abnormal and destructive adaptations to life problems. There may be genetic and chemical tendencies to these disorders.

How to Deal with Mental Illness

Therapy

This refers to intervention by others to provide mental health care. Talking with a friend or a minister, for example, is a form of therapy. At the other extreme is a Freudian-type psychoanalysis consisting of four to five sessions per week and lasting for years. Psychoanalytic technique varies with the particular school, of which there are many. Usually it consists of relaxing on a couch, not facing the therapist, and "free associating" about your feelings, dreams, or past (whatever pops into your conscious mind from the unconscious). Presumably, the analyst can guide one through an insightful therapeutic result. Results are questionable at best—it is probably moot anyway since few can afford it and insurance companies won't pay for it.

Between these extremes in mental health providers are family doctors, professional counselors, social workers, self-help groups, psychologists, and psychiatrists. Does therapy help? Sometimes. According to a survey of *Consumer Reports* subscribers reported in the November 1995 issue, the great majority of responders claimed they were helped to a greater or lesser degree. Apparently, length of treatment was quite important. Those undergoing treatment for longer than six months did better than the short-termers. The type of therapist didn't seem to make much of a difference; all types were successful. The greatest improvement was in those who started out "feeling very poorly," but all groups claimed a degree of benefit in either working out some problems or improving their lives. (Other studies have indicated that similar groups did just as well with time alone.) Psychoanalysis, on the other hand, although reportedly a fascinating and liberating experience, has had quite a mixed critique. It has lost credence and favor as a therapeutic option for the great majority mainly because of the expense, which is far out of the reach of almost all but the wealthy. The results are either spectacular or disastrous, depending upon the critic. In any case, psychoanalysis has declined as a mode of treatment for these reasons. In my own experience, I have not seen any patients who appear to have benefited greatly, although many consider analysis a marvelous learning process.

It would appear that psychotherapy is worthwhile and does help troubled people much of the time. Why? Although the object of therapy may ultimately be to bring insight and acceptance to the patient, this may not happen very often. Sometimes it is enough to have the opportunity to ventilate one's anguish and indecision to someone who will simply hold still and listen. It is too bad that we lonely humans have to pay to have this happen, but that is the way it is too much of the time. Many of us just do not have the support of family and friends who have the time or inclination to fulfill this function. For some, religious faith, meditation, and the like, suffice very well. (Unfortunately, religious cults and other unsavory social groups prey on this need, and are a real hazard in our day and age.)

Medicines (Psychoactive Drugs)

The ancients found that certain herbs, tree barks, weeds, and flowers seemed to settle down their demon-infested cavemates. These protopsychiatrists would prescribe Indian snake root, decoction of hemp, juice of the poppy, eye of the newt, anything that worked to stop the howling. Little could they know that five millennia or so hence Upjohn, Merck, Lilly, and others would do the same for our suffering citizens and make a lot of money doing it. Our species has long sought and found ways to alter our uncomfortable moods.

Psychoactive drugs must, by law, be prescribed by a licensed physician. They are potent mood- and consciousness-altering substances that deserve respect and prudence in their use. Modern psychopharmacy started at the early part of this century with the discovery of the barbiturates (phenobarbital and others); a group of drugs that are calming and hypnotic agents. Barbiturates are still used nowadays, especially as anesthetics (Pentothal® and clones). They do make people sleepy, however, and they are deadly in overdose, which makes them favorite suicide medications. By midcentury newer, milder, and safer calmative drugs were found and given the appellation tranquilizers. Many of these drugs have come and gone in the past forty years.

The class of tranquilizer that has become by far the most popular with both doctors and patients is the benzodiazepines. They are effective in doses that do not cause marked sleepiness and they are far safer than previous tranquilizers. They do not cause as much depression of breathing as do the barbiturates. Fatal overdosage rarely happens, if the drugs are taken alone. Alcohol can be a killer when taken with almost any drug, including these. The benzodiazepine group include long-acting types (especially Valium®, Tranxene®, Centrax®) which last for days, medium acting (Xanax®, Ativan®), which last twelve to fifteen hours, and ultra-short acting (Halcion®). There are reasons and indications for all of these but in general, the medium-acting ones seem to cause less problems. These drugs are not considered addicting, although some patients develop habituation and physical dependence of some degree after long-term use. This is particularly true of the long-acting variety, but it can happen with any one of them. It is best if they are used on only an occasional basis or for a short term (from four to six weeks) during anxiety crises. Slow withdrawal is necessary. Xanax is particularly useful for panic states and episodes. Even though these drugs are generally not very sedating, some caution is required before driving or performing other potentially hazardous activities.

Antidepressants

A funny thing happened on the way to a tuberculosis cure. One of the medications that seemed to help kill these germs (iproniazid) had the peculiar effect of waking up and elating tuberculosis patients, long before the tuberculosis itself was cured. The doctors were amazed to see these chronically ill, debilitated people with tattered lungs get up and literally dance around their beds. Thus was born, in mid–twentieth century, the science of brain chemistry. These strange new drugs seemed to reverse the mental and physical depression of severe chronic illness. There had to be a chemical reason for it. An enormous effort was launched and neurochemistry was born. In the past fifty years our understanding of the chemical processes in the brain that result in happiness, depression, pain relief, and addiction forever altered our lives, not to mention the field of psychiatry. There are brain hormones, called neurotransmitters, which attach to receptors on brain cells and affect our moods. There are stimulating ones such as serotonin and noradrenalin which, when present in adequate amounts, are mood elevating, or antidepressant. There are sedating and pain-relieving ones known as endorphins. These various substances are maintained by enzyme systems which can either lower or raise their levels in brain tissue by enhancing or inhibiting production and utilization. The various classes of antidepressants work by increasing or decreasing the amounts of neurotransmitter activity. Antidepressant drugs are very potent medicines. They have potential serious side effects and their use requires much skill and knowledge by the prescribing physician. Some types, particularly the kind known as MAO inhibitors and the class known as tricyclics (amytriptiline, imipramine) may be deadly if overdosed or used improperly.

The large number and choices of the various psychoactive drugs, each with their own list of side effects, dangers, and advantages, have made treatment somewhat difficult. As a result, there is a new medical specialty known as psychopharmacology which deals solely with the use of these agents, singly or in combination with each other. Usually, primary physicians and psychiatrists will prescribe relatively few of them with which they are familiar and comfortable. The use of these medications, as with any medicine really, represents an experiment with any patient. Everyone is unique and responses are individual as well. Careful and deliberate dosage with close observation is imperative.

The more recent introduction of an apparently safer class of antidepressants, known as the selective serotonin reuptake inhibitors (Prozac, Paxil®, Zoloft®), has raised interesting questions. They tend to cause less grogginess, have fewer side effects, and are far less dangerous in overdose. For these reasons and superior effectiveness for mood elevation, Prozac® and similar drugs have caught the attention and favor of the populace. Literally millions of people have taken one or another of these mood enhancers in what has been called cosmetic pharmacology. Do these drugs enhance one's personality? Do they make the shy person outgoing? These are some of the questions that have been raised. If the answer is "yes," is it necessarily a good thing? The matter has become an ethical, philosophical, and now even a legal matter. Do these drugs, in addition to raising one's spirits, raise one's courage and depress one's inhibitions in a deleterious way? A number of cases of suicide and violent behavior have surfaced and Prozac® has been blamed; notwithstanding the fact that depressed people are more likely than others to commit suicide or behave violently with or without medication. The media and legal professions are having a great deal of play with this. Advocacy groups, one way or another, are fighting pitched battles (for example, drug companies versus Scientology, which has labeled Prozac "the Killer drug"). Scientific investigation of these charges has so far found no merit in them. In my experience, the drugs have some dose-related tendency to cause excitement and hyperactivity in certain individuals; that is, although Prozac, for instance, is marketed in 20 mg capsules, some people do fine on 2 mg and develop overactivity and even anxiety states on larger doses. Here is where skill and individualization in dosing is vital. The range for Prozac has been found by psychopharmacologists to be 2mg to 100 mg per day in different patients!

As far as the philosophical question, "Is mood enhancement meddling with nature or treating an ailment?" I suppose it is both and so is all medical intervention. Clearly it has helped many people feel better, although by itself it has not solved any realistic life problems. On the other hand, if one is able to face one's problems more readily, why not? Some feel these drugs have wrongfully seduced patients away from more meaningful therapy. Maybe so, but insurance companies seem to be keeping people away from therapy more than are the antidepressants. In my view there is a place for both pharmacy and therapy in the area of mental health but the balancing is difficult.

One other matter is pertinent: aside from the considerable cost of these medicines, they all have some potential side effects. They all, for instance, have some depressing effect on sexual desire and potency. There is a long list of other possible (usually mild or infrequent) side effects. Patients should read drug information inserts, though occasionally they can be alarming, and discuss any questions with the doctor.

There are two other types of commonly used psychoactive drugs. First is lithium. This is a chemical salt which is the drug of choice for manic-depressive illness. Maintenance (ongoing) treatment is helpful in the great majority of such patients. Second, there is a whole class of antipsychotic medicines known as the neuroleptics. The first one was Thorazine® but there are many of them now. These are extremely potent blockers of the neurotransmitter dopamine and they have revolutionized the management of schizophrenia and other psychoses. They are the drugs that have made possible the closure of the mental asylums. They should not be used for lesser mental disturbances because they are extremely potent and potentially dangerous.

Alternative Medicine

I previously gave my opinion on this subject, but a few words are in order in this section dealing with mental health. Again, there is no question but that exceedingly valuable chemicals and medicine have been, and are, derived from so-called natural or herbal sources. Research in this area has been, and is, carried out more feverishly than ever since the large drug companies who support such research have noted that this has become an incredibly profitable industry. Indeed some large, legitimate pharmaceutical houses are actually now marketing herbals even though they are not legally (i.e., FDA designated) considered drugs.

A few of these bear mentioning here because they are being marketed for treatment of mental disorders.

St. John's wort, for instance, has been attested to relieve mild depression and anxiety. A chemical called hypericin, which is an ingredient, is thought to be the active principle, but it has not been proven to be so, and the antidepressant chemicals, if present here, have not been found. It seems to be harmless enough, although it may be sunlight-sensitizing.

Kava root is known to be a mild stimulant and muscle relaxant but should not be used with alcohol. Again, the active ingredients are not known.

A few other herbals such as ephedra and borage are known hazards.

And so it goes; ginseng, valerian, ginkgo, and others are being sold for various similar purposes. Most of the time, it seems, without deleterious effects. Okay. But tell your doctor what you are doing. Some naturals are either dangerous in themselves or in combination with other drugs. Watch out!

Drugs of Abuse

There is a wide range of drugs that are abused.

Opiates (morphine, heroin, codeine)

These are all derivatives of the opium poppy. Opium itself was used in prehistoric times as a folk remedy but was outlawed sooner or later in most societies because of the serious dangers of associated addiction. Opium and its derivatives have a long, fascinating history of political and socioeconomic intrigue and dirty dealing, which continues to this day. The opiates work via the same brain chemistry principles as outlined before. They attach themselves to the brain cell receptors that accept our own natural painkillers, the endorphins. The effect, however, is much stronger and longer lasting and the "high" so induced is the basis for addiction in those so prone (some people more than others; why, as yet, is a mystery). To the addict, the drug is more essential than food, as necessary as air, and he concentrates all thoughts and feelings on the need to procure it. What was taken for pain relief or for pleasure has become an inexorable tyrant. The crude opium, solidified poppy juice, is a complex mixture of chemicals known as alkaloids. The first was morphine, discovered in the eighteenth century by the German chemist Setulieus who must, in balance, be considered a great benefactor of mankind, as well as a Pandora. Morphine and similar alkaloids are still the most important drugs used for the control and relief of severe pain. The medical uses of the opium alkaloids are many and important. The nonmedical uses have had tragic consequences.

Coca and Cocaine

The ancient pre-Incan Indians found the leaf of the Andean coca plant to provide comfort and stamina during stressful times, such as high-altitude labor. These half-frozen, half-starved men chewed the leaves with a bit of soda lime to release the active alkaloid, cocaine, for absorption. A German physician, Dr. Scherzer, brought this plant back to Europe in 1840. Researchers isolated the pure alkaloid shortly thereafter. Interestingly, this new miracle drug was touted for treatment of morphine addiction! Among the experimenters was Dr. Sigmund Freud who in the 1880s had his own struggle with morphine and codeine addiction. He was fortunate enough to escape these shackles, and was also instrumental in the finding that cocaine is a marvelous local anesthetic; that is, by simple application to the membranes of the nose, eyes, and mouth, it can numb them. It is still used for surgical anesthesia on these organs. Unfortunately, it has become a favorite substance for abuse. If cocaine is sniffed, smoked, swallowed, or injected, it is a strong and addicting narcotic. It is the drug of choice of the poor—it is grown by the poor (Andean farmers) and used by the poor. Between these two are the criminal rich and corrupt officials.

Amphetamines

Another class of excitatory and euphoria-producing substances is the amphetamines, derived chemically from the ancient Chinese ephedrine herb (ma-huang). This class of drugs was synthesized in the early twentieth century by the

Japanese-American pharmacologist Dr. H. Takamine. These drugs were considered miracle substances; antidepressants, stimulants, and appetite suppressants. Currently the commonly used appetite suppressant, phentermine, is actually derived from the amphetamines. They were in common medical use until the 1960s, when they began to be abused. Not only were they addicting, they (particularly methamphetamine and dextroamphetamine, Dexedrine®) were even more so than cocaine. They attach themselves to the same neurotransmitter receptors as cocaine. In overdose they produce severe hyperactivity and paranoia and in withdrawal, severe depression. They are now strictly regulated for occasional medical use (for example, in narcolepsy, a disease marked by severe somnolence and, paradoxically, for use as a calming agent for hyperactive children). Most of the amphetamines being abused these days are illegally manufactured.

Marijuana (hash, weed, pot, hemp, reefer)

This is an ancient herb which, when smoked or eaten, is a potent intoxicant. Whatever one's opinion of this natural drug, it has remained popular throughout the ages. It even has useful and legitimate medical indications (for example, for glaucoma and nausea of cancer treatment). The basic ingredient is the chemical tetrahydrocannabinol (THC) which varies only in amount of the product inhaled or ingested. The drug is long lasting, persisting in the tissues and blood for about three weeks. It causes euphoria but also depresses reflexes and inhibitions. Whether or not it leads to addiction to other drugs is debatable, but legally it is considered a malignant substance to be suppressed. Medically speaking, we know that smoking pot in large doses is as bad for the lungs as tobacco; usually, it is not inhaled in as large amounts or as constantly. It is just as dangerous as alcohol when it comes to driving. The question of addiction, per se, has not been answered. However, it is not as addicting as opiates or cocaine. Should it be as permissible, legally, as alcohol? This is a debatable question. Both drugs are known to have potential dangers to reproduction; they have fetus-damaging potential and marijuana has been demonstrated to have chromosome-altering properties. My own feeling is that marijuana and alcohol are both hazardous substances and require much self-control to avoid harm. There has been only dismal failure when governmental control has been attempted. Abuse of these substances has flourished and so have the criminal exploiters. At the very least, I believe that use of the weed should be decriminalized. I would love to see some of the vast sums used to purchase it go toward the national debt instead of to the dealers. As for legalization and government licensure and taxation of recreational drugs in general, an excellent argument can be made for this. We have clearly lost the war on drugs and we continue to waste more and more of our resources waging this dubious battle. Our prisons are overcrowded with far more victims than suppliers. We are enriching an apparently untouchable criminal class, while drug use seems to be increasing, particularly among the young. If illicit profit is eliminated, perhaps much of this tragedy would stop. Official regulation and distribution would at least help prevent turning our deprived youth into criminals who steal and kill to get a "fix." Funds derived from licensure could also be used for appropriate treatment, or at least some control of addiction. There appears little hope otherwise of controlling this evil. If something has been done about tobacco, why not other substance abuse?

Alcohol

It has been said that if alcohol were discovered now it would take ten years to get through the FDA, and it would be sold by the teaspoonful to a grateful nation and world by giant drug companies at five bucks a dose. It would, after another ten years, go generic and the price would fall to $3.50. After a while and much argumentation and pleading, it would go over-the-counter and be sold for $2 per half-teaspoonful. Of course, by now basement laboratories would have discovered the secret and would distribute it on street corners for $1 per teaspoon. Users, of course, would be severely punished and the prison industry would flourish. (Alcohol is easily made in prison cells.)

Consumption of alcohol is widely accepted in almost all societies as a normal practice. It is even a regular event in nonhuman societies; birds and bears are well known to ingest fermented berries when available. Human society has known and used alcohol since Neolithic times. It has been treasured and considered a boon to some, yet it is recognized that in excess it is undesirable and deleterious. There is controversy, however, about what constitutes use and abuse and how to tell them apart. There are many definitions of alcoholism and alcohol abuse. To some, deviation from a societal norm is abuse, whereas others require demonstrable physical harm or addiction to alcohol. The World Health Organization states that alcoholism exists "when the consumption . . . exceeds the limits accepted by his culture . . . at times deemed inappropriate . . . or intake becomes so great as to injure health or impair social relationships." The American Psychiatric Association adds "evidence of psychologic dependence or need to continue daily functioning" . . . "continuous or frequent episodes of intoxication may also be present." Addiction to alcohol is characterized by extreme tolerance and physical symptoms of withdrawal such as the DTs (delirium tremens, a serious neurologic breakdown with shaking, hallucination, and delusions). Tolerance may be so great that an individual may appear sober with sky-high blood alcohol levels.

The causes of alcoholism are also fraught with controversy. The genetic propensity is there, at least statistically, with sons of alcoholics at far greater risk, as are identical twins (rather than fraternal ones). The roles of social factors and stress are less clear but of obvious importance. Alcohol is a temporary problem solvent, not a solver. Many alcoholics themselves (particularly AA spokespersons) insist that there is an actual chemical imbalance that drives a person to drink and alcoholism; that the only solution to the problem is total and permanent acceptance of the defect and total and permanent abstinence with the constant help of fellow alcoholics and a higher being. This, in short, is the basis of the famous twelve-step program which, incidentally, has been adapted by all sorts of self-help groups.

The medical hazards of alcoholism are many. Intoxication itself, aside from the immediate danger to oneself and others, can lead to acute poisoning, not to mention early withdrawal symptoms, hangover, tremulousness, nausea, sleeplessness, and even cardiovascular problems in those who are prone. Chronic use may lead to severe nutritional deficiencies, brain and nerve disease, and heart and liver disease. The social and interpersonal damage is monstrous (illustrated in the marvelous and accurate films *Lost Weekend*, *Days of Wine and Roses*, and *Leaving Las Vegas*). As a physician, I can say that alcoholics are the most challenging and frustrating patients. Frequently lovable, they often simply cannot be brought out of their suicidal ways much of the time. It is a common experience that the AA approach has been the most effective. Long-term treatment, often marked by frustrating relapse, is necessary. Drugs such as Antabuse® (disulfiram) may be tried but they are very dangerous if a patient goes "off the wagon" while taking them.

Can people drink safely? Of course they can. I've already mentioned the French Paradox. (However, alcoholism and cirrhosis is quite common in France.) There is the possible risk factor of total abstention, at least in the Framingham statistics. Can an alcoholic become a controlled drinker? A few people think that this is possible, but the most serious alcoholics, the AA group, scoff at such a suggestion. Can one live without alcohol? Sure, ask any observant Muslim or Mormon. They do fine. Incidentally, I inquired of a Mormon physician friend of mine why his religion, a Christian one, proscribed alcohol since the Bible does not. His answer was that it is for strictly social reasons. The Mormons treasure family values far more than they do the transient warmth of the juice of the grape. For you? You'll have to decide for yourself.

Violence

This is considered a social aberration, but I wonder. I find, with my biological orientation, little surprise in the apparently increasing incidence of aggressive destructive behavior. After all, nature has never stopped being "red in tooth and claw." As much as we hate to admit it, the drive-by shooting, the Serb-Bosnia neighborhood massacre, the Rwandan-Hutu-Tutsi affair, and the murderously crowded rat cage are phenomenologically similar.

Assuming that violence potential exists as part of our makeup, are there internal factors that modulate the expression of this behavior? It appears to be so. There are areas in the animal brain which, upon stimulation, produce uncontrollable rage. Drugs which suppress our inhibitions (alcohol, PCP) permit outrageous violent behavior in otherwise apparently civilized persons. Does our male sex have anything to do with this? Apparently so, for the virilizing male steroid hormones, testosterone and its derivatives, do affect behavior and aggressiveness. It is quite suggestive that much violent crime seems to be testosterone driven; for example, the awful statistics involving teenage boys and steroid-infused athletes.

The usefulness of this knowledge, unfortunately, is limited. Castration of the male criminal (once a legal option, at least in sex offenders) is not a humane punishment. However, we can try to prevent or at least try to convince our young athletes to lay off the steroids. Not only do they have serious side effects, they also can make one sterile.

Insomnia

Insomnia, a common difficulty, is not in itself a mental disorder, but it may be a vexing problem with multiple potential causations. Worry, anxiety, depression (whether neurotic or reality based) certainly are prominent causes, as is physical disease. Chemical causes include overuse of stimulating drugs such as caffeine, or certain antidepressants. Alcohol withdrawal can cause associated sleeplessness.

Do we need sleep? Apparently so. Sleep is divided into two types: REM (rapid eye movement) sleep and non-REM. The REM type is associated with dreaming and many active autonomic functions, penile erection, and muscle jerking and twitching. The non-REM is a quiet type with variable degrees of depth. The non-REM comprises about 80 percent of sleep. Normal adult sleep usually lasts about seven hours with a range between four and ten hours. Sleep not only serves to recharge our psychic batteries (sleep deprivation may lead to severe nervous symptoms), but many physiologic functions and hormonal cycles depend upon a sleep-wake schedule. For instance, growth hormone is secreted by the pituitary mostly during sleep.

Can't sleep? Check your habits. Caffeine is present in substances other than coffee; for instance many soft drinks, tea, and chocolate. Avoid these and other stimulating foods at bedtime. Cut down your intake of alcohol, particularly colored alcoholic beverages. Whiskeys, brandies, and red wines contain substances called congeners which, in addition to giving color and flavoring, may also contain stimulating chemicals. Check your regular medications for side effects (ask your doctor). If you clearly have emotional problems that are responsible, seek help or therapy. Try relaxation techniques: a warm bath, soothing reading, or counting sheep. (A friend of mine tries self-hypnosis, or trying to fig-ure all names that begin with a certain letter. I tried it myself and ended up get-ting up and going to an encyclopedia. Not a good technique for the compulsive.) Finally, if nothing else helps, see your doctor. Physical disease should be excluded and if done so, I think it is perfectly acceptable to use, on occasion, a mild medium-acting tranquilizer such as Ativan or Xanax or a mild nonbarbiturate sleep inducer such as Ambien®. Suppression of REM sleep by barbiturates or other older sleeping medications is not good; it may lead to withdrawal night-mares and other possible physiologic problems.

DR. DASHE'S TIPS FOR HEALTH MAINTENANCE

1. Men generally have more difficulty expressing their emotions and talking about their problems. This is why suicide and violent reactions are more common in men than in women. Don't let your ego keep you from getting help if you are in emotional pain.

2. Mild depression, or "the blues," is not uncommon and will go away with time and activity, especially if it is causal (death of a loved one, losing your job).

3. Chronic depression is not so easily dealt with and might require extensive psychological therapy as well as medication.

4. As more is discovered about chemical deficiency in the brain, the ability to use medications to restore balance becomes a more viable alternative.

5. Alcohol and drugs are not good ways for dealing with emotional problems; both can only complicate and worsen matters for you.

6. Once again, a balanced lifestyle will help you deal with life emotionally; exercise, good nutrition, and activity will make life more palatable in most cases.

7. Psychotherapy by lay or professional persons may be helpful and effective in alleviating mental suffering.

Chapter 14

GETTING THERE—MAKING IT (AGING)

Now that you have read and heeded all my advice and lived the good, moderate, prudent, healthful life and had the requisite luck, here you are, aging. Aging? Comes to mind, Oliver Hardy's statement to Stan Laurel "Another fine mess you've gotten us into now." (You know you are chronologically challenged, when no one you mention this to seems to know who Laurel and Hardy are.) Nervously you notice a certain ambivalence about aging; in yourself as well as in others. It is little comfort to realize that the alternative is not particularly desirable either. I will attempt to describe, if not define, the aging process, discuss some of the latest theories of causation, discuss some of the particular health problems of aging, and conclude with some upbeat observations that don't often come to mind.

What Is Aging?

I was about five years old when, falling asleep one night, I heard some nice soothing motherly voice singing the words to "Taps" (the "lights out" bugle call of the military). The song ended with the line "God is nigh." I didn't know what "nigh" meant, but I knew that God was an old man with a white beard. I mistook nigh for the number nine. Ergo, to my immature imagination: 1) God was nine years of age, and 2) at age nine, a long time away to be sure, one became old. Well, it seemed reasonable to me, but when I passed the age of nine I had to put off the aging process to a later date, and I find myself still doing the same thing. Being old is something far away. So much for what we think; old age is clearly something that happens in the future and to somebody else.

Scientifically, aging seems to be the culmination and merging of pathways of decline in our physical and social lives. All living things are subject to this process. Much speculation goes on in our thinking species as to the reasons and causes for aging, senescence, and finally mortality.

Our bodies consist of trillions of cells functioning quietly to keep us alive. These cells all produce chemicals (hormones to regulate our metabolism, antibodies to fight off invaders, enzymes to digest our food, and so on). These exquisite and complex activities and processes are themselves regulated by enzymes that are produced from the DNA molecules of our cells; little blueprints that we have inherited from our parents. If defective DNA is passed on, we may have conditions known as congenital defects. The effects of these might range from miscarriage to lifelong disability. Even in health, however, this complex machinery can break down, interfering with cell function and even causing cell death. Our cells die and are replaced constantly; that is, those that are capable of replication. Some of our cells, particularly in the central nervous system, are nonreplaceable and when lost are gone forever. (Recent evidence in lab rats, at least, seems to show that some nervous system cells may regenerate, but persist only if they are put to use by physical or mental exertion.) When the DNA templates themselves are damaged or altered, this is a far more ominous and dangerous development. The change not only affects the cell in which it occurs, but also all the descendants of the defective cell. If the chemical product of that cell is altered, the consequences to the body can be serious and a disease state produced.

Damage to cellular DNA may occur from many different sources; chemicals, radiation, or other nefarious influences. Fortunately, there are DNA repair enzymes patrolling each inch of our DNA chains (about 6 feet of chain in each cell). We have natural defenses to chemical aggressors. For instance, harmful oxidant chemicals may be neutralized by antioxidants in our food. (Whether added antioxidants such as beta-carotene or vitamin E supplements help this process is controversial.) The longer we live, the more attacks to our cellular integrity and defense we absorb. It seems reasonable, as with any unceasing siege, that our defenses will break down. It is well known that cancer is associated with abnormal changes in the genes that control our cellular growth. The incidence of cancer increases with age, so we can reasonably make the inference that our DNA defenses have been breached finally by too many assaults. Things, after all, do wear out.

Can we have any say in this matter? Yes, we can, in some obvious ways. We can choose to avoid or curtail noxious poisons such as smoking, alcohol, and excesses of almost any kind. Avoiding excess radiation is more difficult. Every time we fly to another city, we get as much radiation from cosmic rays as a chest x-ray. A flight to Europe is about equal to a full mouth x-ray. The molecular biological explanation of aging, which I have described, comes from the fertile mind of Professor Bruce Ames of the University of California at Berkeley. There are other concepts and theories, of course, but this seems to be the simplest common denominator. Ames, quoted and explained eloquently by Dr. James Trefil in the *Smithsonian* claims, sensibly, that it is impossible to avoid all the risks of living. Try to avoid the major known ones: "Don't smoke . . . drink moderately . . . eat a balanced diet with lots of fruits and vegetables . . . and . . . just do what your mother told you."

Theories on How to Live Longer

Exercise

Can regular exercise lengthen life expectancy? Such claims have been made but evidence is only suggestive. It is true that the fit and vigorous withstand disease better than the sedentary and obese, but actual years of extended longevity have not been proven. Regular exercise has many other advantages, so why not?

Obesity versus Leanness

There seems to be little doubt that excessive obesity (greater than 20 percent) is associated with early development of serious disease (arteriosclerosis, diabetes, cancer) and decreased longevity. The question of the benefit of being underweight or even being somewhat malnourished arises. Some scientists, particularly Dr. Roy Walford of the UCLA School of Medicine, are vociferous in this claim, although they have no human studies to prove it. Not many people, I think, would volunteer for such an experiment in deprivation, even if life extension could be guaranteed. Dr. Walford points out many instances in nature where the slim outlive (and outrun) the better nourished. (Skinny rodents do outlive fat rats.) His personal regimen consists of a vegetarian diet several hundred calories short of his predicted requirement, accompanied by supplemental necessary nutrients (vitamins). He certainly appears to be a fine, slim, and vital human specimen. Dr. Walford proposes reasonable life expectancy into the early hundreds with such a spartan regimen. There are theoretic reasons for giving Dr. Walford's theory credence. The ingestion of potentially toxic substances are cut considerably, and it is well known that one's metabolic rate slows with caloric deprivation and hormone production decreases; nature's way of prolonging life under dire circumstances.

Longevity Drugs

Hardly a month passes without an apocalyptic announcement that a new drug has arrived that will rejuvenate the fading and hold off the angel of death. As far as I know, neither of these promises has ever been kept, but some interesting observations have been made. The use of the female sex hormone, estrogen, has resulted in a considerable improvement in the health of postmenopausal women. The incidence of such killers as arteriosclerosis and osteoporosis in such treated women has plummeted and with this, longevity enhanced. Can the same be claimed for testosterone use in men? Not quite. For one thing, testosterone production in men persists well into the seventh and eighth decades. Second, there is some evidence that testosterone supplementation may enhance tissue (muscle and bone) integrity and libido and the feeling of well-being in the aging male.

The downside may be that of enhancement of atherosclerosis via deleterious effects on blood cholesterol. Certainly, no one has yet shown any effect on longevity, one way or another. Other natural human hormones, notably growth hormone and, more recently, an adrenal gland androgenic (male-type) hormone with the off-putting name dehydroepiandrosterone (DHEA), have also been touted as the answer to the problem of aging.

Growth Hormone

This has been well demonstrated to be necessary for the growth of immature mammals to the adult state. Past this, function in the adult is unknown. Given to a normal mature subject, there is some increase in protein utilization and muscle, bone, and tissue growth. As a matter of fact such growth, if uncontrolled (as in the case of acromegaly, a disease caused by a growth hormone–producing pituitary tumor) is not only undesirable but catastrophic, with disfiguring enlargement of the face and extremities. Diabetes, arthritis, and arteriosclerosis may also result. Administration of growth hormone also has an exorbitant cost of about $800 per month. DHEA is cheaper, and as yet unregulated; but as is usually the case, it seems to be too good to be true. I doubt its claims and urge caution.

Melatonin

There are many anecdotes about the benefits of melatonin. It is a hormone of the pineal gland, important in our sleep and wake cycles; but studies on effects, both good and bad, have never been done, nor is manufacturing or dosage regulated.

Vitamins, Antioxidants, Hormones, Amino Acids

Remember tryptophan? There were a number of unexpected deaths before this "wonder" amino acid was removed from the market.

To date, the search for life-lengthening drugs, hormones, and other measures goes on. Human life expectancy has increased enormously since the dawn of history, at least threefold. Most of the credit must go to public health measures rather than medical science per se, but immortality eludes us.

Some final observations: Married men live longer than single, divorced, or widowed ones. I can only surmise that caring for and having a caring wife in itself is something to live for, not to mention that having a partner usually abets nutrition, hygiene, and sexuality. Also, there seems to be little question that the old adage "use it or lose it" applies not only to artistic skill, but to life itself.

Health Problems of Aging

What Happens When a Man Ages?

Aging starts at the moment of conception. One's potential is no greater than at that time. Think of it; out of that single-celled creature develops trillions of other unique and variously specialized cells, all combining and functioning together to create a person. In a way, it's all downhill from there, depending upon how you look at it. Actually, it's more like a roller-coaster ride, because our various organs and functions develop, fulfill their functions, and when finished in their purpose, wane. Our growth, for instance, is uphill until our second decade; from then on, we tend to shrink. Our muscle strength and agility peaks in the third decade; from then on, it diminishes. On the other hand, our ability to understand and control our lives develops with the years, if we and circumstances permit it. In the past, our revered sages were all senior citizens.

Heart and blood vessels. Things wear out, and our hardest-working muscle, the heart, is no exception. Cardiovascular disease is by far the greatest cause of death in the aged. I've already discussed the preventive measures to preserve your heart as long as possible.

Cancer. Again, a disease group that increases in incidence with time; the second greatest cause of mortality. There is a lot more that can be done now in prevention, detection, and treatment, but I believe malignant disease will always be with us in one form or another.

Diseases of the central nervous system. By the time we reach puberty, the brain and central nervous system are fully developed, anatomically and mechanically. Their precious cells cannot be replaced when lost (see page 242); they have no ability to divide and replicate as do some other organs (liver, bone marrow). This, perhaps, is why a sudden destruction of a portion of our brain because of clot or hemorrhage is known as stroke. The ancients who coined the term recognized the frequently devastating result, and considered this the stroke of a vengeful deity. Things are a bit better now and we do have some promising modes of management and rehabilitation, but it's a severe, if not devastating event. How to avoid it? Take care of yourself, particularly your blood pressure and cholesterol, and stop smoking. Stroke and smoking are intimately related.

Parkinson's disease. The area of the brain that regulates the coordination of our muscle activities is known as the extrapyramidal system. The smoothing out of muscle activity is elegantly regulated by this incredible computerlike mechanism which is faster than any man-made electronic system. If damaged, muscles cannot work in proper unison; this creates what we know as tremulousness or, alternately, spastic stiffness. There are many causes of such extrapyramidal damage. These usually, but not always, occur in later life. They may include viral disease, stroke, toxic effects of some drugs used to treat psychosis, and some "designer drugs" of abuse. A genetic basis for Parkinson's is rare. Victims of this disease are frequently afflicted with a peculiar stiffness of muscle and facial expression and a repetitive-type of tremor of the hands. There may be a crippling, unstable gait. Little could be done in previous years, but now there are some effective medicines and some types of brain surgery which are ameliorative. Still, it is a relatively uncommon disease compared, for instance, to cardiovascular disease.

Dementias, including Alzheimer's disease. Deterioration of intellectual functioning while consciousness is otherwise present define these sad situations. There are many causes including injury (for example, from boxing), infection (such as syphilis), toxicity (severe alcohol or drug abuse), severe nutritional deficiencies, brain tumor, multiple strokes, psychoses, and many others. The type that has gotten much media publicity, particularly since President Reagan's dramatic announcement, is Alzheimer's disease, which is a mysterious affliction of unknown and probably multiple causes. The diagnosis is frequently made by exclusion; that is, when no other reason can be found for the symptoms. The typical case begins with some memory loss and selective amnesia with an apparently normal social facade. A family member will note problems, although the victim may appear normal to the casual observer. Gradually, the patient's difficulty becomes obvious and incapacitating (for example, getting lost, losing valuables). Communication ability begins to deteriorate after two or three years and further abilities such as dressing and caring for oneself gradually and variably diminish. The age of onset is usually seventy to eighty, but may be younger (rarely). The incidence rises with age, and some form of dementia occurs in 10 to 15 percent of the population over the age of eighty-five; accounting for most of the nursing home population in this country. Women are more frequently affected than are men, but this is probably because they tend to live longer than we do.

Much research is being done to find a cause, and therein a prevention or treatment for this tragic malady. It is known that genetic predisposition may be a factor in some, but not all, cases. A recent long-term study of an order of nuns suggested that intellectual defects may actually be present early on, even in youth in later-affected subjects. Pathological studies of brain tissue in Alzheimer's victims generally show placques of a peculiar protein substance called amyloid, as well as tangles of fibers of brain cells, a veritable scarred wasteland.

As previously stated, the diagnosis of Alzheimer's disease is usually by exclusion. There are no specific tests to establish the diagnosis, only tests that may find other causes for dementia. Neurologic centers usually will perform a variety of sophisticated, expensive examinations which frequently come up with a blank, again leading to a diagnosis of Alzheimer's. Tests include various complex blood chemical examinations to rule out the far less common metabolic causes of dementia. Brain scans, especially MRI, are useful to detect causes such as multiple small strokes which leave characteristic scars, and the uncommon but treatable late-onset normal pressure hydrocephalus. This disorder may be marked by dementia and more specifically, episodes of falling and bowel and bladder incontinence. If caught early and treated with a plastic tube shunt procedure, which relieves the fluid buildup in the brain, all the symptoms may be reversed.

Most commonly, however, no treatable disorder is found and the Alzheimer's patient must be cared for in a sympathetic and supportive manner, with special attention paid to nutrition and other medical needs. The prognosis is invariably negative but the care and comfort given should not be. There are no specific medications at this time that relieve the dementia, although a few have been touted. They have not been effective in most cases, as far as I know. Tacrine (Cognex®) and doneprezil (Arecept®) are the only drugs approved by the FDA for treatment and the results are discouragingly modest. Some have suggested that NSAIDs or aspirin may possibly act as a prophylactic agent, as it does in arteriosclerotic disease, but the evidence thus far is slim. In any case, prophylactic aspirin is in common use for other reasons and should, in my view, be taken by most people who are able to tolerate it.

There is little that can be said that is encouraging about dementia except that if you are reading this now, the odds are much in your favor that you will not be a victim. This is a great fear of patients over the age of forty, who see their personal physicians because of lapses of memory. These lapses are the norm for all of us over that age for a number of reasons. First of all, the older we get the more there is to remember. Our memory banks are so laden that retrieval takes time. We tend to be distracted by too many things in these days of high-stress living. We may have psychological blocks for certain things. It is true, too, that we are losing brain cells to wear and tear over the years, although the myriad connections that make up our memory capacity are able to bypass shutdown cells with alacrity. Anyway, that's another reason why we have reference libraries and computers.

Sight and hearing. These senses, too, are affected by the passage of time. Starting at the age of thirty-five, the lenses of our eyes begin to stiffen so that we are unable to make rapid adjustments to focal changes of distance. This condition, known as presbyopia (presby = elder, opia = vision), causes the previously perfect youthful eye to strain with near vision (we can't adapt fast enough). Reading glasses are required; simple magnifying lenses costing a few dollars at your local store work fine. Of greater concern is the increasing incidence of cataracts (opacification of the lens of the eye) and glaucoma (an increase of pressure in the eye associated with visual loss). These defects (possibly genetic) are easily detected at periodic (every two years) eye checkups, either by an ophthalmologist (M.D.) or an optometrist (O.D.). The latter professionals are able to detect these common diseases, although they are not allowed, by law, to treat them. They do well with refraction for glasses; anything more complicated requires an M.D. ophthalmologist. Treatment of glaucoma is usually medical, using various eye-drops, although occasionally surgery is necessary (using the laser). This instrument has revolutionized treatment in ophthalmology and many heretofore hopeless situations, such as retinal hemorrhages from diabetes mellitus or other causes, may be successfully managed with this space-age beam. Treatment of cataracts also has been wonderfully improved, even during my medical lifetime. Surgical removal of a cataract used to be a major surgical procedure with almost a full week of hospitalization. The patient was frequently forced to lie motionless, head held firmly between sandbags, for several days. It was a terrible experience and after the surgery, vision was frequently impaired by the absence of the removed lens and the required adjustment between the eyes. Occasionally, because of this, doctors opted to wait until both eyes were practically blind before one cataract could be removed. Now, the operation is completed in a matter of minutes. The cataract is usually simply liquefied, removed, and a new plastic lens implanted. The patient is up and around immediately and vision restored almost at once, with both eyes functioning together. Miraculous! The procedure has gotten so simple and routine that it has, I fear, become too commonplace in a way. Most older eyes have some lens opacity, but this does not mean that immediate surgery need be done. For one thing, surgery is surgery, no matter how simple it may be, and there are always some risks. If a patient can see well enough to drive, read, or watch TV, there is no urgency for cataract removal. It can be done at a later time if necessary, without further loss of vision by simply waiting.

Hearing, on the other hand, is a different matter. Most hearing loss associated with aging is of the nerve deafness variety and is not amenable to surgery. The other major category of deafness, the conduction variety, is far less common and is usually caused by congenital or other type of disease, scarring, or rigidity of the eardrum and/or its bony connections to the inner ear and auditory nerve.

Conduction deafness may be amenable to surgery by particularly skilled and specialized ear surgeons. Nerve deafness, at least at this point in time, is not, and sound amplification devices (hearing aids) may be the only alternative. A few warnings are in order. There are many well-advertised hearing aid stores. They will be more than willing to sell you a device without going to the expense of performing a legitimate hearing evaluation. Chances are you will regret such a purchase and have an expensive piece of unusable hardware around to remind you of your mistake. Get a referral to a qualified audiologist from your physician. These specialists can properly test your hearing and advise you on the type of appliance that will be best for you and your pattern of hearing deficit. It is far better to start using these devices early on, rather than waiting until the deficit is totally incapacitating. The adjustment is thereby gradual and much more effective, rather like gradual accommodation to darkness versus being plunged from a brightly lit room into a dark cave. There are other important considerations, and expert guidance is highly desirable.

Other problems of the aging man. One point should be remembered—the elderly person is a survivor. He has proven resilient to the diseases that limit existence. The longer you live, the longer you live. To quote a tough lady, actress Bette Davis, on the subject: "Aging is not for sissies." There are some recurrent themes in the complaints of aging male patients. Many have to do with security and financial concerns, particularly regarding the presence of ageism in the workplace. For example, talk to any TV or motion picture writer over the age of thirty-five, and they'll tell you it's difficult to find work. The same applies to many professions and activities. Worries about medical insurance and long-term care are frequent. The natural decline in strength and agility and the stiffness and achiness that comes with age is aggravating, as are the changes seen in the mirror. Creases, jowls, and pot bellies are depressing, particularly to the more narcissistic men among us.

These ubiquitous feelings are handled one way or another, at the worst, by increasing alcohol or drug use, an expanding geriatric problem. There are those who try to do something about the various inequities; the plastic surgeon may iron or laser the wrinkles, suck the handles, dejowl the chin, plug the scalp, and so on. Others may simply ignore or learn to abide the burdens of time and look to the marvelous opportunities, sights, and sounds previously unavailable to them. Yet others, perhaps luckier in a way, must continue to work to survive, luckier because work keeps us vital, if not chronologically young. It is important, in my view, to be involved in something, exercise, diet, exploration, education, volunteering, anything to keep active.

Statistically, the potential life span increases with each passing year. Children born now have a life expectancy of about seventy-five years. If you are already seventy-five, you have beaten the odds and probably have another ten to go. The downside of this is obvious. There is gradual decline in strength and function of all of our systems. However, with the help available to us, medical and otherwise, these health problems are made bearable, if not curable. Your physician is clearly a key person at this time of life; that is, when you need a physician. Our healthiest people are the ones who see the doctor least.

Death and Dying

I feel that I must discuss what I alluded to at the beginning of this book: a healthy death. As a physician, I have made it my own personal philosophy to avoid telling people how to live. Advice yes, commandment no. I feel similarly about death. I tell no one how to die. I also feel it my duty to give a patient all the information I reasonably can about his condition and prognosis. No doctor is a licensed or certified prophet and no one can give more than an educated guess about the number of days left to a patient. As a mortal human as well as a man of responsibility to others, I have taken certain personal steps that I consider vital. I urge all my responsible patients, aging or not, to consider doing the same.

I refer to proper instructions to your doctor and your next of kin or significant or responsible other. You must make known your own desires with regard to your medical care, well before your final days. There are choices, and you have legal rights in the matter. These rights are best designated in the form of a living will as well as a "Durable Power of Attorney for Health Care." These legal papers are easily available from your attorney or even from stationery stores. They are invaluable if you are unable to make your final decisions because of illness or mental incapacity. I am not, by this, urging euthanasia, a currently highly charged, emotional issue. Dr. Jack Kevorkian, who may be thought of as the John Brown of the euthanasia wars, has brought the matter to a head in recent years. Without commenting about Dr. Kevorkian's style, I can say frankly that the majority of physicians conscientiously believe in euthanasia, of the passive type at least; that is, with the permission if not instruction of the patient or his designated agent, various life-supporting measures may be withheld or withdrawn. This is now legal in most places. What is not realized is that many, if not a majority of physicians, are authorized to provide pain relief to an individual suffering from a terminal lethal illness, even if this cuts short his life. Whether or not you want to call this active euthanasia is immaterial. Hippocrates's second instruction to his physician disciples was "relieve pain" (the first, of course, was "do no harm"). Clearly, a physician has some choice in this matter, too, so you should find out if your doctor's ethics correlate with your own, and act accordingly.

Finally, before I leave this sad but necessary subject, I would like to share with you an observation. "Death with dignity" is an expression used to describe the admirable exit of an individual who has maintained his decorum throughout his last days. This cherished state is superseded only, in my view, by "death with grace" in which the dying individual manages to help those around him to maintain theirs.

What's Good About Aging?

Well, you don't need a haircut or a manicure as often, do you? You don't sweat as much, so you probably smell better. Your mild, short-term memory lapses are more than compensated for by superior judgment based upon experience. You need less sleep. You have built up immunity to many diseases over the years and your allergies diminish. You enjoy simple things more, including a lovely day or a tree. You've slowed down enough to actually see things. You have time now (assuming that, like most folks over sixty-five, you've retired) to do things that are pleasant and leisurely, which you could never do before. If you're still married, you've probably settled most of your hot disputes. You probably get along better with your wife. Even interest and pleasure in sex don't diminish much; 90 percent of people over age sixty still enjoy it. The aging in our society, increasing in number as they are, have more political and economic clout. They vote, more than any other group. It's kind of nice to get those discounts: movies, hotels, museums, airfare. Inexpensive opportunities for travel, education, and cultural broadening open up amazingly. Such organizations as Elderhostel provide magnificent experiences for the older population. The opportunity is there, and it is up to you to take advantage of it. Prepare for it before retirement. There is nothing sadder than the man who takes retirement with nothing to do. The illness and even mortality rates for such unfortunates is shockingly high.

Alfred Tennyson wrote a poem on the subject, *Ulysses*, which to me should be the anthem of the aging man. An excerpt:

> Old age hath yet his honour and his toil . . .
> Some work of noble note may yet be done
> Not unbecoming men that strove with Gods . . .
> Tho much is taken, much abides; and tho
> We are not now that strength, which in old days
> Moved earth and heaven, that which we are, we are,
> One equal temper of heroic hearts,
> Made weak by time and fate, but strong in will
> To strive, to seek, to find, and not to yield.

DR. DASHE'S TIPS FOR HEALTH MAINTENANCE

1. The causes of senescence and mortality are not known but appear to be inherent in our genetic makeup.

2. Longevity research and theory is a burgeoning area rife with speculation; although life expectancy continues to climb, immortality is still beyond our reach.

3. Vision and hearing problems are common to aging. Major improvements in detection and treatment in the area of eye disease have helped overcome many problems. Hearing problems can be helped with a hearing aid.

4. The major and most difficult problems of aging, such as Alzheimer's disease and other dementias and stroke, have to do with loss of brain function. As research continues, more will be done to deal with these brain-related maladies.

5. There are some definite advantages to aging, including the peace of mind that comes with experience and more reverence for time and its use. The aged are survivors, and don't forget the discounts.

6. Dying is an unpleasant chore, but you can do it with grace and comfort. Make sure your family has an idea of your wishes should you become incapacitated and unable to make your own decisions.

7. Although not a medical matter, you should always be prepared for your eventual demise.

Chapter 15

TO BE A MAN

The changes in our society, particularly since the end of World War II, have produced staggering stresses upon us all. But this book deals with men, so I have emphasized our troubles rather than those of women. Actually the troubles are shared, so this attitude is admittedly somewhat artificial. A woman's menopausal depression affects her family greatly, for example. But, though I may be accused of sexual prejudice, I must point out the singular tensions placed upon us and our gender in the past five decades.

We were born into an authoritarian and paternalistic ethos, but now the father has been assaulted and demoted, even demeaned by that same society, its media, and the very real socioeconomic milieu. The destruction in so many ways of the traditional family is both the cause and the result of this confusing muddle.

Prior to World War II, the family was an economic unit by necessity. The father was understood to be the strong one who brought home the bacon and protected the women and children. Women, and children too, had their duties and responsibilities, but life would not be life without father. Divorces were few compared to the decades that followed. The family was united and goal oriented; the goal being survival of all concerned, hard work for everyone. Ageism was unheard of. Grandma and grandpa worked until they couldn't anymore, but they were supported and revered as long as they lived. How simple it all was.

So what has happened? Whether it was good or bad, this basis of our civilization has crumbled, it would appear, most everywhere. I cannot and will not presume to say why. I cannot place the blame on women, men themselves, or any particular group. Religionists point to the loss of religious fervor or belief; I rather think this is more a result than a cause of the problem. Blame, anyway, is irrelevant.

I realized early on that teenage sociopathy had one common thread—an absent father. As a young Air Force physician, one of my duties was to medically and psychiatrically examine airmen who were to be dishonorably discharged for one offense or another. Notably, it had to be a major offense. The group, disparate as it was, had one common property—an absent or abusive father. Destruction of the functional family has always been the most effective facilitator of demoralization and slavery of a population, such as in the antebellum south. The destruction of the "father" system, combined with the sexual revolution, Vietnam, Watergate, and so on, has apparently undermined our societal structure. The cumulative effects of this, and the pressures exerted by the women's movement, gave the weakened male ego further feelings of emasculation and frustration. This should by no means be construed to be an antifeminist statement. I believe strongly in the necessity for equality of the sexes in most of the ways for which women are fighting. I also believe in and cherish the differences between us. I think the paternalistic society erred greatly in ascribing strength to the male and weakness and subservience to the female. This error has in no short measure been responsible for the perceived attack upon us by women—an unfortunate assumption on our part.

Women have been and are as strong as men. Their strength, although manifested differently than ours, is no less potent. Together both sexes complement one another to create the formidable species that we are. There is no advantage in having one sex be the master of the other. Not only is it a counterproductive concept, it is both unreal and inane. Equal pay for equal work applies not only to the job market, but also to all aspects of life. This equality is the yin and yang of our existence and must not be unbalanced. Thus, if we feel that our maleness is threatened, if we are disappointed, let us ask ourselves, who appointed us in the first place? Let us cease this whining of victimization and be responsible for ourselves, our children, and our own actions. Even if, for whatever reason, our marriages must terminate, our paternal duties, moral, fiscal, and symbolic must not. Let understanding and acceptance of our need for the complementary strength of our significant others be the source of our augmented manhood. In other words, let us grow up and be real men.

But this is not enough. Acknowledging those artificial and erroneous threats is an important step, but not the only one. Being a man has other requirements. First and foremost a man needs to have a sense and confidence in his own worth as a productive human being. He cannot do this unless he does some form and amount of work, no matter if manual or mental, paid or volunteer. Without this, we men are subject to despair, depression, and potential disastrous acts of violence, addiction, or other sociopathy (often noted as diseases of the twentieth century). A man must also try to be a decent person and maintain friendships and social intercourse with other decent persons. One can't ignore the scoundrels all around us but we don't have to emulate or cultivate them, nor antagonize them either, especially on a freeway where a gesture or look can draw gunfire. Other key indicators of decency are courtesy, a neglected virtue in this cyber-electronic age, and enlightened selfishness (the "golden rule"). Enlightened selfishness means that actions that are responsible, openhearted, and kind are at the same time self-serving and may bring a like response from others. This is a concept that requires some thought, but it is the ethical basis for all the humanistic religions and is the best bet for our survival and that of our children in a tough world.

We might no longer have fathers to emulate or to make sure that we do these things, but if we do these things *we* will be good fathers, not to mention good people. And we will be men. And healthy ones at that.

Suggested Additional Reading

Alternative Care

Alternative Medicine: Expanding Medical Horizons. Washington, D.C., U.S. Government Printing Office, 1994, #NH 94-066.

Boyle, T.C. *The Road to Wellville*. New York, Viking Penguin, 1993.

Herbal Roulette. *Consumer Reports*. November 1995, pp. 698–705.

Drugs

Brown, D. *Smoke and Mirrors: The War on Drugs and the Politics of Failure*. Boston, Little, Brown & Co., 1996.

Exercise

Getting in Shape. *Consumer Reports*, January 1996, pp. 14–29.

Levin-Gervasi, S. *Back Pain Sourcebook*. Los Angeles, Lowell House, 1996.

General

The Harvard Medical School Health Letter, Harvard University Press.

Thomas, L. *The Medusa and the Snail: More Notes of a Biology Watcher*. New York, Viking Press, 1979.

Trefil, J. *How the Body Defends Itself from the Risky Business of Living*. Smithsonian, 26:42–49, 1995.

University of California at Berkeley Wellness Letter. P.O. Box 420149, Palm Coast, Fla. 32142.

Mental Health

Davidson, F.G. *Alzheimer Sourcebook for Caregivers*. Los Angeles, Lowell House, 1996.

Does Therapy Help? *Consumer Reports*, November 1995, pp. 734–739.

Nutrition

Federal Dietary Guidelines for Americans, Consumer Information Center, Dept. 378-C, Pueblo, Colo. 81009.

University of California at Berkeley. *Wellness Encyclopedia of Food and Nutrition.* Berkeley, UC Press, 1996.

Weight Control: Do Diet Pills Work? *Consumer Reports.* August 1996, pp. 15–17.

Sexuality

Annotated Bibliography of Books on Sexuality. Publications Department, SIECUS, 130 W. 42nd St., Suite 550, New York, N.Y., 10036-7802.

Comfort, A. *The Joy of Sex: A Cordon Bleu Guide to Lovemaking.* New York, Pocket Books, 1987.

Zilbergeld, B. *Male Sexuality.* New York, Bantam, 1993.

Glossary

Acid blockers: antihistamine-like medicines, such as cimetidine, that prevent the formation of acid by the stomach

Acid pump blocker: powerful medicines, such as omeprazol, that prevent cellular manufacture of acid in the stomach

Acidosis: an excess of acid substances in the blood

Acne rosacea: a chronic reddening and inflammatory skin condition, primarily affecting the face

Acne vulgaris: common type of acne, usually affecting adolescents

Acromegaly: disease of excess growth of tissues caused by abnormal secretion of growth hormone

ACTH: adreno-cortical-trophic hormone. The pituitary secretion that stimulates the adrenal gland to produce its hormones

Acupuncture and moxibustion: ancient Chinese medical treatment which involves placement of a needle in the skin with or without heating with a burning herb (moxa)

Adrenal glands: endocrine glands lying over the kidneys, source of adrenal steroids and epinephrine (adrenaline)

Adrenaline: trade name of epinephrine; hormone of the medulla (center) of the adrenal gland

Aerobic: requiring air or oxygen

Agoraphobia: morbid fear of open places

AIDS: acquired immune deficiency syndrome, caused by the human immunodeficiency virus (HIV)

-algia: suffix meaning pain

Alkaloids: natural alkaline, organic plant compounds, frequently useful medically but also frequently drugs of abuse (morphine, heroin, cocaine)

Allergen: agent capable of inducing a state of allergy

Allopathy: modern scientific medicine

Allopecia: hair loss

Allopecia areata: patch of circumscribed hair loss, frequently of the scalp

Alpha hydroxy acid: fruit acids used in dermatology to stimulate skin rejuvenation

Alternative medicine: medical practices and disciplines other than allopathy

Alveoli (alveolus): cavity, depression, pit, or cell, such as in the lung

Alzheimer's disease: dementia of unknown origin associated with characteristic pathologic changes in the brain

Amphetamine: synthetic stimulating drug related to ephedrine and epinephrine

Amylase: an enzyme which converts starch to sugar

Anabolism (anabolic): tissue building

Anaerobic: life sustained in the absence of oxygen

Analgesic: pain reliever

Androgen: male steroid hormone, from testicle or adrenal gland

Androsterone: androgenic (male) steroid hormone produced by the adrenal gland

Angina pectoris: chest and arm pain due to lack of oxygen to the heart muscle

Angiography: radiographic visualization of a blood vessel via injection of liquid which shows on x-ray

Angioplasty: reconstruction of a blood vessel, usually via a balloon catheter threaded into the vessel

Antacid: a medicine that relieves or neutralizes acidity

Antibiotic: a chemical usually derived from a fungus or plant that can suppress or kill micro-organisms

Antifungal: an antibiotic that can suppress or kill a fungus

Antihistamine: a medicine that neutralizes or prevents the effects of histamine, used for the treatment of allergies

Anti-inflammatory: a drug or chemical that prevents or ameliorates inflammation

Antinausea: medicine, such as Dramamine, used to prevent or treat nausea and vomiting

Antioxidant: chemicals such as vitamins C and E and beta carotene, which allegedly prevent destructive oxidative processes

Antipyretic: fever-treating medicines, such as aspirin, acetaminophen

Antiseptic: germ-killing chemical

Antitussive: cough suppressor

Anal sphincter: muscle of the anus

Aorta: main artery of the body

Aphrodisiac: stimulator or enhancer of sexual desire or performance

Apocrine: glands that secrete externally, such as sweat or oil glands

Appendix (vermiform): a small blind sac attached to the right side of the colon (cecum)

Arteries, arterioles: blood vessels that carry oxygenated blood from the heart to the tissues

Arteriosclerosis: thickening and narrowing of the inner lining of the arteries, usually by cholesterol and/or calcium; hardening of the arteries

Artificial tears: protective eyedrops that prevent drying of the eyes

Asbestos: fibrous silicon, damaging to the lungs when inhaled

Asthma: shortness of breath due to spastic narrowing of the bronchial tubes

Audiologist: a specialist in hearing disorders

Auscultation: listening through the stethoscope

Autonomic: automatic functions, especially of the nervous system (for example, sweating)

Axial skeleton: bones of the head and trunk (spine, neck, and skull); the vertical axis of the body

Barrett's esophagus: chronic inflammatory precancerous condition of the lower esophagus

Basal carcinoma: a common type of skin cancer

Beriberi: vitamin B-1 deficiency disease

Bibliotherapy: treatment by education, especially reading

Bile acid: a digestive component of bile that is secreted by the liver

Bile pigments: breakdown products of hemoglobin secreted in the bile by the liver

Bipolar disorder: alternating depression and euphoria; a mood disorder

Blackhead: a blocked oil gland

Bladder: the urine reservoir in the pelvis

Dislocation: disarrangement or displacement of a joint

Diuretic: a chemical promoting excretion of urine

Diverticulosis (-itis): pouches or sacs opening from the inside of the colon; -itis = inflammation of same

DNA (deoxyribonucleic acid): genetic material of chromosomes

DTs: delirium tremens, acute insanity due to alcoholism

Duodenum: first portion of the small intestine, leading from the stomach

Dupuytren's contracture: scarring of the palm with deformity of the fingers

Dysentery: an infectious diarrheal disease due to various microorganisms

Dyspepsia: indigestion

Echocardiogram: sound-wave pictures of the heart

Edema: watery swelling of the tissues

Ejaculation: semen emission

Electrocardiogram: graphic recording of electric currents of cardiac activity

Embolism: a clot or plug blocking a blood vessel coming from a distant source (for example, the leg)

Emphysema: chronic disease marked by breaking down of the walls of lung tissue

Endocrine: glands of internal secretion

Endocrinology: medical study of endocrine glands

Endorphins: natural pain-relieving and pleasure-enhancing brain neurotransmitter chemicals

Endoscopy: visualization of various internal structures via a fiberoptic scope

Epiglottis: a flap, valve-like structure that protects the glottis (windpipe opening) during swallowing

Epinephrine: adrenal medulla "fight or flight" hormone

Esophagus: swallowing tube

Euphoria: feeling of well-being, exaltation

Exocrine: glandular secretion via a duct (for example, pancreas enzymes enter into the digestive tract via the pancreatic duct)

Expectorant: chemical that promotes loosening and expectoration of mucus

Extensor: a muscle that bends to extend or straighten a limb

Femur: thighbone

Fever: temperature above normal

Fibula: outer and smaller of the two bones of the lower leg

Flatulence: intestinal gas

Flatus: expelled intestinal gas

Flexor: a muscle which bends or flexes a joint

Flu: a general term for a respiratory or gastrointestinal infection, not to be confused with true influenza

Foreskin: sliding sleeve of skin that covers the head of the penis; also called the prepuce

Fracture: a broken structure, usually a bone

FSH: follicle stimulating hormone of the pituitary gland

Fugu: Japanese blowfish with a very poisonous liver

Fundoplication: surgery to repair a weak lower esophageal valve

Fungicide: a drug or chemical that suppresses or kills fungus

Furuncle: a simple boil of the skin

Gallbladder: bile storage sac of the liver

Gallstones: stones forming in bile, usually within the gallbladder

Gastrin: hormone of the gastrointestinal tract (especially the stomach) that stimulates acid secretion

Gastrointestinal: pertaining to the stomach and intestines

Gastroscope: device (usually fiberoptic) for internal visualization of the stomach

Genital warts: warts of the genital and anal area caused by human papilloma virus, sexually transmissible

Genitourinary: pertaining to the kidney, ureters, bladder, and genital organs

GERD: gastroesophageal reflux disorder

Germ plasm: reproductive material

Glans penis: head of the penis

Glaucoma: an eye disease, associated with increased pressure within the eye, which may lead to blindness

Glottis: opening of the larynx (voice box) and windpipe

Glucagon: an endocrine hormone of the pancreas that stimulates elevation of the blood sugar

Goiter: enlargement of the thyroid gland

Gonadotropins: reproductive stimulating hormones of the pituitary glands

Gonads: the sex glands, testes, or ovaries

Gonorrhea: a sexually transmissible disease caused by the gonococcus germ

Gout: a metabolic disease associated with elevated blood uric acid levels and recurrent attacks of arthritis

Graves's disease: a form of overactivity of the thyroid gland

Grip(pe): influenza; name erroneously given to any upper respiratory infection

Growth hormone: a pituitary hormone which stimulates growth of the body; also called somatotrophin

H2 blocker: see acid blocker

Hair follicle: skin depression from which a hair grows

Hallucinations: perceptions of objects and sensations that are unreal

Hashimoto's thyroiditis: allergic or autoimmune chronic inflammation of the thyroid

HDL: high density lipoprotein cholesterol; "good" cholesterol

Heartburn: a burning chest sensation due to dyspepsia

Helicobacter pylori: bacteria implicated in causation of chronic peptic ulcer

Hemoglobin: red oxygen-carrying pigment of red blood cells

Hemophilus ducreyi: germ causing chancroid, a venereal disease

Hemoptysis: coughing up blood

Hemorrhoids: varicose veins of the rectum and anus; also called piles

Hepatitis: inflammation of the liver

Hernia: rupture; protrusion of an organ or structure through the wall that contains it

Herpes simplex: viral blister disease, usually recurrent

Herpes zoster: shingles, chickenpox virus causing a rash and pain along the course of a sensory nerve

Hiatus hernia: protrusion of stomach into chest

Hirsutism: abnormal hairiness

Histoplasmosis: fungal disease, usually of the lungs

HIV: human immunodeficiency virus; viral cause of AIDS

Homeopathy: an alternative medical discipline founded by Dr. Samuel Hahnemann

Hormones: natural chemical messengers between tissues and glands

Human papilloma virus: virus that causes human warts

Hydrocephalus: increased fluid in the chambers of the brain

Hydrocortisone: adrenal steroid hormone with many important metabolic and anti-inflammatory functions

Hyperglycemia: high blood sugar level

Hyperhidrosis: excessive sweating

Hyperparathyroidism: overactivity of the parathyroid glands with overproduction of parathyroid hormone and elevated calcium blood levels

Hypertension: elevated blood pressure

Hyperthyroid: overactivity of the thyroid gland with overproduction of thyroid hormone

Hyperventilation: overbreathing, increased frequency and depth of breathing

Hypoglycemia: low blood sugar level

Hypothalamus: primitive part of the brain that controls the endocrine system and many automatic functions

Hypothermia: low body temperature

Hypothyroid: underactivity or underfunction of the thyroid gland

Ileocolic valve: valve between the small intestine (ileum) and large intestine (colon)

Ileum: third and last part of the small intestine

Immunization: rendering immunity, usually through a form of vaccine or antitoxin

Incontinence: inability to control bladder or bowels

Indigestion: inability to digest food comfortably; dyspepsia

Infection: invasion of tissues by bacterial or viral microorganisms

Inflammation: a reaction in tissues caused by irritation or infection marked by swelling, redness, pain, and heat

Inflammatory bowel disease: diarrheal diseases of the intestines such as regional enteritis and ulcerative colitis

Influenza: a severe viral infectious respiratory disease; the "grip(pe)"

Inguinal canal: pathway of the sperm cord through the groin and abdominal wall

Inguinal hernia: rupture of the inguinal canal

Insulin: endocrine hormone of the pancreas which allows blood sugar to enter tissue cells for metabolism

Interstitial cells: cells of the testes that produce male hormone (testosterone)

Iontopheresis: electric current treatment of skin

Irritable bowel syndrome: oversensitivity of the lower intestinal tract marked by cramping, alternating diarrhea and constipation, and increased mucus in the stools

-itis: suffix meaning inflammatory

Jaundice: yellowing of the skin due to retention of bile pigment

Jejunum: second part (midpart) of the small intestine

Kidney: main blood-filtering organ that removes wastes and produces urine for disposal from the body

Kidney stones: crystalline bodies formed in the kidneys, usually from calcium salts or uric acid

Korotkov sounds: sounds produced by the blood pressure cuff compressing an artery

Laxative: medicine that stimulates bowel action

LDL: low density lipoprotein cholesterol; "bad" cholesterol

Legionella: microorganism that causes Legionnaire's disease, a pneumonia

Leptin: an obesity-preventing hormone (recently discovered in rats and other mammals)

Lesion: a wound, injury, or abnormal change in tissue

LH: luteinizing hormone; a gonadotropin or sex gland stimulating hormone of the pituitary

LHRF: luteinizing hormone releasing factor; a hypothalamic hormone that regulates pituitary sex hormone production

Libido: sexual desire

Liniment: a liquid applied to the skin for soothing or stimulating purposes

Lipase: fat-digesting enzyme

Lipoprotein: a blood protein that carries fat, particularly cholesterol

Lithium: an element which is used as a medication for treatment of manic-depressive disease

Liver: the largest abdominal organ with multiple functions including digestion processes, blood filtration, detoxification and excretion of wastes, and manufacturing of many necessary body chemicals

Lumbar: the lower five vertebral bodies between the thoracic spine and the sacrum

Lymphogranuloma: a venereal disease caused by chlamydia

Malabsorption: inability of the intestine to digest and absorb ingested food

Malaise: feeling of illness

Mania: excessive enthusiasm or excitement

Manic depressive: a psychosis marked by alternating bouts of mania and depression

MAO inhibitor: monoamine oxidase inhibitor; an antidepressant medication

Marijuana: cannabis sativa; leaves and flowers of the hemp plant used as a mild narcotic and stimulant

Masturbation: self-stimulation of the genital organs

Megavitamin: excessive dose of a vitamin

Melanoma: a tumor arising from a pigmented mole

Meniscus: a crescent-shaped body, usually refers to the knee cartilage

Microsurgery: surgery performed through small apertures or via microscopic instrumentation

MRI scan: magnetic resonance imaging; tissue visualization via magnetic wave stimulation

Mucus: a viscous liquid secreted by numerous glands, especially bronchial or intestinal; has both cleansing and lubricating functions

Murmur: an abnormal sound produced by passage of blood through a roughened vessel or valve

Mycobacterium: a genus of bacteria causing some human diseases, especially tuberculosis and leprosy

Myocardial infarction: death of cardiac muscle due to loss of blood supply

Naturopathy: an alternative system of health care

Nephritis: inflammation of the kidney

Neuroendocrine: hormonal interactions between brain and endocrine glands

Neuroleptics: drugs used to treat psychoses (for example, Thorazine®)

Neurological: pertaining to the nervous system, brain, and spinal cord

Neurosis: nonpsychotic emotional disorders characterized by anxiety, depression, obsession, and psychosomatic symptoms; also called neuropsychosis

Neurotransmitter: central nervous system hormones, especially of the brain

Norepinephrine: an important neurotransmitter hormone; also an adrenal hormone

NSAID: nonsteroidal anti-inflammatory drugs (aspirin, ibuprofen, and many others)

Obesity: excessive bodily fat deposits

Occult: hidden or unrealized, such as occult fracture of the wrist

Omnisexual: sexual preference that is general and unlimited

Ophthalmoscope: instrument for visualizing the interior of the eye

Opiates: the crude narcotic mixture derived from the opium poppy, *Papaver somniferens*, from which the narcotic alkaloids morphine and codeine are derived

-osis: suffix meaning a condition of disease, usually chronic

Os penis: the bone of the penis present in certain mammals

Osteoarthritis: degenerative or wear-and-tear arthritis; chronic joint wear and deformity with variable inflammation

Osteopathy: an alternative health discipline, now mostly incorporated into allopathic medicine

Osteoporosis: loss of bone substance

Otitis: inflammation of the ear, usually the middle ear

Otoscope: instrument for visualizing the eardrum and canal

Ovaries: female gonads

Oxidants: chemicals that cause oxidation of tissues and cells

Palpation: examination by feel

Palpitation: awareness of irregular or unusual beating of the heart

Pancreas: abdominal organ with dual endocrine (regulation of blood sugar) and exocrine (digestion) functions

Pancreatitis: inflammation of the pancreas

Panic: irrational, overwhelming fear leading to illogical feelings and beliefs

Papilloma virus: virus that causes warts

Paranoia: feelings or delusions of persecution

Parathyroid: endocrine gland imbedded in the thyroid which control calcium metabolism; there are four

Parkinson's disease: a degenerative brain disease characterized by tremor and rigidity

Pediculosis: infestation with lice (body, head, or pubic)

Pellagra: vitamin deficiency disease, caused by a lack of niacin

Penometer: device that measures nocturnal erections

Pepsin: a stomach enzyme that breaks down protein

Peptic ulcer: a lesion of the esophagus, stomach, or duodenum caused by stomach acid and pepsin

Percussion: examination, particularly of the chest, by tapping with fingers

Pericarditis: inflammation of the external lining of the heart (pericardium)

Pericardium: membrane lining the heart

Peripheral blood vessels: arteries, capillaries, and veins coming from and returning to the heart

Peristalsis: propelling, wavelike movements of the intestinal tract

Peritoneum: lining of the abdominal cavity

Peritonitis: inflammation of the peritoneal cavity

Peyronie's disease: a fibrous deformity (bending) of the penis

Pharyngitis: inflammation of the pharynx, usually infectious

Pharynx: the throat cavity between the glottis, esophagus, and nasal passages

Pheromone: a chemical released by an animal which may affect the feelings or behavior of another animal, especially sexual attraction

Phimosis: narrowness of the foreskin preventing it from drawing back over the glans

Phobia: unreasonable fear or dread

Piles: hemorrhoids; varicose veins of the anus or rectum

Pitiriasis rosea: scaly red skin rash caused by a fungus plus allergy

Pituitary gland: a major endocrine gland located at the base of the brain

Plantar wart: a wart on the sole of the foot, usually at a pressure point

Pleurisy: inflammation of the lining (pleura) of the lungs

Pneumococci: genus of bacteria that is a common cause of pneumonia and other serious infections

Pneumonia: an infection of the lung tissue

Polyp: an outgrowth or swelling from a mucous membrane

Polypharmacy: overutilization of multiple drugs or medicines

Portal circulation: the separate blood system of the intestinal tract via the liver

Premature ejaculation: uncontrolled early ejaculation during or before intercourse

Presbyopia: inability to rapidly focus on near objects, caused by aging of the eye muscles

Priapism: persistent penile erection

Proctology: medical specialty dealing with large intestinal problems

Prolactin: pituitary hormone; one of the gonadotropins and lactation-inducing hormone in the female

Prolactinoma: tumor of the pituitary gland that secretes prolactin

Prostate gland: semen production gland surrounding the beginning of the urethra at the base of the bladder

Prostatitis: inflammation of the prostate gland

Protease: enzyme that digests proteins

PSA: prostatic specific antigen; substance produced only by prostatic tissue that is detectable in the blood

Psoriasis: chronic inflammatory red patchy rash, occasionally associated with arthritis

Psychoactive drugs: medications that affect mood and/or thinking

Psychoanalysis: a system of uncovering unconscious thoughts and mechanisms devised by Sigmund Freud and his followers

Psychopath: mentally disturbed individual apparently devoid of social conscience or responsibility

Psychosis: a mental illness characterized by impaired contact with reality, occasionally marked by delusions and hallucinations (for example, schizophrenia)

Psychosomatic: physical illness caused by or affected by emotional factors

Psychotherapy: treatment of mental disorders

Ptyalin: a sugar- and starch-digesting enzyme of saliva

Pulmonary embolism: blood clot that travels to and lodges in a pulmonary artery, usually from a leg or pelvic vein

Pyelonephritis: infection of the kidney

Pyloric valve: sphincter valve between the stomach and duodenum (first part of the small intestine)

Radioiodine: radioactive isotope of iodine, used for diagnosis and treatment of thyroid disease

Radon: radioactive gaseous element, a suspected cause of lung cancer

Rectum: last portion of the colon ending at the anus

Reflex: an involuntary response to a stimulus (for example, twitch of a muscle when a tendon is tapped)

Regional enteritis: Crohn's disease; an inflammatory bowel disease, usually involving the terminal portion of the small intestine (ileum)

REM sleep: rapid eye movement sleep associated with dreaming and penile erection

Renal colic: cramping severe pain usually caused by passage of a kidney stone

Retina: light-receptive layer of the eye

Rheumatoid arthritis: inflammatory systemic disease, autoimmune in nature, affecting joints and other organs

Rhinophyma: acne rosacea of the nose, causing bulbous red swelling

Rotator cuff: muscles, tendons, and ligaments which form the cuff covering and surrounding the shoulder joint

Roughage: high-fiber-content foods, especially vegetables and grains

Saliva: secretion of the salivary glands of the mouth; a lubricating, digestive, mild antibiotic substance

Salivary glands: glands producing saliva (parotid, submaxillary, and submental)

Salt: sodium chloride; common table salt and the major salt of body tissue

Scabies: a mite that causes severe itching and a transmissible skin rash

Scaphoid bone: a wrist (carpal) bone particularly prone to occult fracture

Schizophrenia: a severe psychosis characterized by flat and inappropriate mood regression and paranoia

Sciatica: pain due to irritation of the sciatic nerve which extends from the buttock to the foot

Scrotum: skin sac that holds the testicles

Scurvy: vitamin C deficiency disease

Sebaceous glands: apocrine glands producing oil called sebum, secreted directly onto the skin

Seborrhea: chronic irritation of the sebaceous glands

Sebum: oil and wax produced by the sebaceous glands

Semen: fluid produced by the prostate gland, the carrier of spermatozoa upon ejaculation

Seminal vesicles: semen reservoir

Seminiferous tubules: tubules of the testes lined with Sertoli cells which manufacture spermatozoa

Serotonin: a stimulatory neurotransmitter

Sertoli cells: cells lining the seminiferous tubules which manufacture spermatozoa

Shin splints: pain in the anterior legs usually associated with exercise

Sigmoidoscopy: visualization of the lower 60 to 70 cms of the colon via a flexible fiberoptic scope

Signs: objective evidence or clues of disease

Sippy diet: multiple feedings of milk and cream, formerly used as an ulcer diet and treatment

Sitz bath: hip bath; old-fashioned medical term for sitting in a small tub of hot water

Small bowel: midintestine consisting of three sections: the duodenum, jejunum, and ileum in that order; also called the midgut

Sociopathy: antisocial behavior; a lesser form of psychopathy

Spermatic cord: cordlike structure from the scrotum to the groin containing the sperm duct (vas deferens), blood vessels, muscle, and ligaments

Spermatozoan: a sperm cell

Spirochete: type of bacteria which may cause disease (for example, syphilis)

Splenic flexure syndrome: left chest pain caused by gas in the colon

Sprain: an overstretching or tearing of a ligament

Sprue: a diarrheal disease caused by allergy to gluten (nontropical) or possibly a virus (tropical)

SSRI: selective serotonin reuptake inhibitor; a type of antidepression medication (for example, Prozac®)

Sternum: breastbone

Steroids: a type of organic compound related to cholesterol; a name given to cortisone and its derivatives or male hormone derivatives

Stool softeners: medication that softens stools, usually a detergent

Streptococci: a type of bacteria that may cause disease (for example, strep throat)

Stricture: a narrowing of a structure usually caused by scarring

Stroke: a sudden blockage of blood to a part of the brain, usually caused by a clot or hemorrhage, causing severe symptoms such as paralysis or sensory loss

Sunscreen: a lotion that protects the skin from the damaging rays of the sun

Symptoms: subjective feelings of disease

Syndrome X: a hypothetical cluster of medical disorders consisting of hypertension, insulin resistance, and elevated blood sugar, insulin, and triglyceride levels resulting in arteriosclerosis

Syphilis: a venereal disease

Systolic blood pressure: blood pressure (upper number) registered at the time the heart contracts, or beats

Tendon: a structure connecting a muscle to a bone

Tennis elbow: bursitis of an elbow tendon

Testes: male gonads

Tetany: muscle spasm, particularly that due to low blood calcium

Thoracic: pertaining to the chest portion of the body

Thorax: the structure between the abdomen and the neck

Thyroid: shield-shaped endocrine gland in the neck that regulates metabolism

Thyroxin: the hormone of the thyroid gland (true name is levothyroxin)

Tibia: shinbone; major bone of the lower leg

Tonsillitis: inflammation (usually infection) of the tonsils of the pharynx

Tophi: uric-acid-containing skin bumps, usually on ears and hands

Trachea: breathing tube

Tranquilizer: a calming or sedating drug

Tricyclics: a family of antidepressants

Triglycerides: a form of fat composed of three fatty acids combined with a glycerol molecule

TSH: thyroid stimulating hormone; a pituitary hormone that regulates thyroid function

Tuberculosis: an infectious (usually respiratory) disease caused by the germ *Mycobacterium tuberculosis*

TURP: transurethral resection of the prostate; removal of a portion of the prostate through the penis

Ulcerative colitis: an inflammatory bowel disease characterized by bloody diarrhea and systemic symptoms

Ultrasound: sonar used in medicine for visualization of certain organs (for example, gallbladder, heart)

Ureteral calculi: kidney stones that pass down into the ureter and to the bladder

Ureters: the tubes leading from the kidneys to the bladder

Urethra: the tube leading from the bladder to the outside

Uric acid: a product of cell metabolism that is excreted in the urine

Uvula: the fleshy flap in the back of the throat hanging from the soft palate

Vaccination: immunization by injection of a portion of an infectious microorganism

Vagus nerve: an internal nerve that supplies the gastrointestinal tract, among other structures

Valley fever: the disease, usually respiratory, caused by the fungus coccidioides, first discovered in the San Joaquin Valley of California

Varicose veins: swollen, distended, tortuous veins, usually due to vein-valve failure

Vas deferens: sperm duct leading from the testes through the inguinal canal to the prostate

Vascular: relating to blood vessels

Vasectomy: cutting or removal of a portion of the sperm duct

Vasopressin: hormone of the hypothalamus and the posterior pituitary that permits the body to conserve water

Veins, venules: blood vessels that return blood to the heart

Vertebra: the 33 bony segments that make up the spinal column, 7 cervical, 12 thoracic, 5 lumbar, 5 sacral (fused into 1), 4 coccygeal (fused)

Virilization: masculinization due to action of male hormone

Viscera: internal organs

Warts: benign external tumors caused by papilloma virus

Wheezing: noise caused by spasm of the bronchial muscles, narrowing the tubes

Whitehead: a blocked sweat gland

Index

Page numbers in *italics* refer to illustrations in the text.